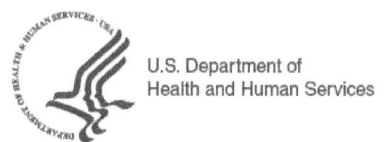
U.S. Department of
Health and Human Services

I0493682

2008 Physical Activity Guidelines for Americans

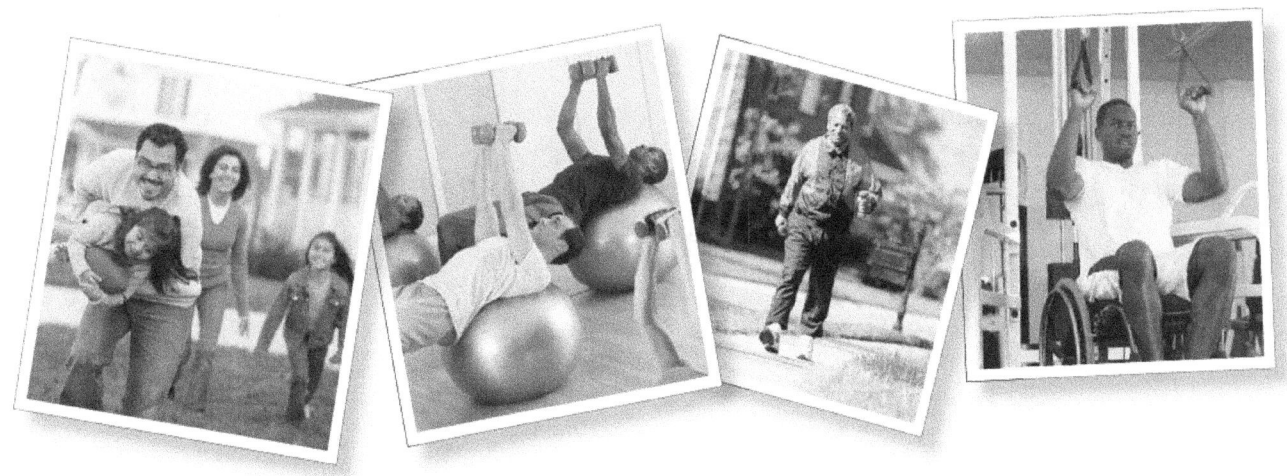

Be Active, Healthy, and Happy!

www.health.gov/paguidelines

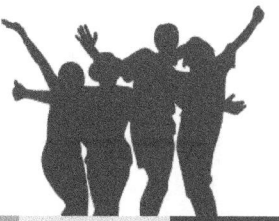

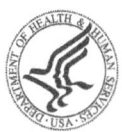

I am pleased to present the 2008 Physical Activity Guidelines for Americans, the first comprehensive guidelines on physical activity ever to be issued by the Federal government. This document is intended to be a primary source of information for policy makers, physical educators, health providers, and the public on the amount, types, and intensity of physical activity needed to achieve many health benefits for Americans across the life span. The good news is that these guidelines are achievable and can be customized according to a person's interests, lifestyle, and goals.

This document is based on the report submitted by the Physical Activity Guidelines Advisory Committee, a group comprising 13 leading experts in the field of exercise science and public health. The committee conducted an extensive review of the scientific data relating physical activity to health published since the release of the 1996 Surgeon General's Report on Physical Activity and Health. I want to thank the Committee and other public and private professionals who assisted in creating this document for their hard work and dedication.

Along with President Bush, I believe that physical activity should be an essential component of any comprehensive disease prevention and health promotion strategy for Americans. We know that sedentary behavior contributes to a host of chronic diseases, and regular physical activity is an important component of an overall healthy lifestyle. There is strong evidence that physically active people have better health-related physical fitness and are at lower risk of developing many disabling medical conditions than inactive people.

Prevention is one of my top priorities. Although physical activity is clearly vital to prevention, it is easy for many of us to overlook. These Physical Activity Guidelines for Americans provide achievable steps for youth, adults, and seniors, as well as people with special conditions to live healthier and longer lives.

Sincerely,

Michael O. Leavitt

Acknowledgments

The U.S. Department of Health and Human Services (HHS) would like to recognize the efforts of the Physical Activity Guidelines Steering Committee that oversaw the work of the Physical Activity Guidelines Advisory Committee and the Physical Activity Guidelines writing group: Rear Admiral Penelope Slade Royall, PT, MSW (Office of Disease Prevention and Health Promotion; Director, Secretary's Prevention Priority); Captain Richard P. Troiano, PhD (National Institutes of Health; Physical Activity Guidelines Coordinator and Advisory Committee Executive Secretary); Melissa A. Johnson, MS (President's Council on Physical Fitness and Sports; Physical Activity Outreach Coordinator); Harold W. (Bill) Kohl III, PhD (Centers for Disease Control and Prevention (CDC); Physical Activity Science Coordinator until October 2007); and Janet E. Fulton, PhD (CDC; Physical Activity Science Coordinator beginning October 2007).

The Department is grateful for the contributions of the HHS scientists and staff who participated in the Physical Activity Guidelines writing group that developed and created this document: David M. Buchner, MD, MPH (chair); Jennifer Bishop, MPH; David R. Brown, PhD; Janet E. Fulton, PhD; Deborah A. Galuska, PhD, MPH; Commander Julie Gilchrist, MD; Jack M. Guralnik, MD, PhD; Jennifer M. Hootman, PhD, ATC; Melissa A. Johnson, MS; Harold W. (Bill) Kohl III, PhD; Sarah M. Lee, PhD; Kathleen A. (Kay) Loughrey, MPH, MSM; Judith A. McDivitt, PhD; Denise G. Simons-Morton, MD, PhD; Ashley Wilder Smith, PhD, MPH; Wilma M. Tilson, MPH; Captain Richard P. Troiano, PhD; Jane D. Wargo, MA; Gordon B. Willis, PhD; and the scientific writer/editor, Anne Brown Rodgers.

The Department also gratefully acknowledges the work conducted by the 2008 Physical Activity Guidelines Advisory Committee. Their extensive review of the scientific literature on physical activity and health and their committee deliberations are summarized in the *Physical Activity Guidelines Advisory Committee Report, 2008*. The Committee's report provided the basis for the *2008 Physical Activity Guidelines for Americans*. The Advisory Committee consisted of William L. Haskell, PhD (chair); Miriam E. Nelson, PhD (vice-chair); Rod K. Dishman, PhD; Edward T. Howley, PhD; Wendy M. Kohrt, PhD; William E. Kraus, MD; I-Min Lee, MBBS, ScD; Anne McTiernan, MD, PhD; Russell R. Pate, PhD; Kenneth E. Powell, MD, MPH; Judith G. Regensteiner, PhD; James H. Rimmer, PhD; and Antronette K. (Toni) Yancey, MD, MPH.

The Department also acknowledges the important role of those who provided comments throughout the Physical Activity Guidelines development process. Finally, the Department appreciates the contributions of numerous other departmental scientists, staff, policy officials, and the external peer reviewers who reviewed the *2008 Physical Activity Guidelines for Americans* and provided helpful suggestions.

Contents

2008 Physical Activity Guidelines for Americans Summary

Being physically active is one of the most important steps that Americans of all ages can take to improve their health. The *2008 Physical Activity Guidelines for Americans* provides science-based guidance to help Americans aged 6 and older improve their health through appropriate physical activity.

The U.S. Department of Health and Human Services (HHS) issues the *Physical Activity Guidelines for Americans*. The content of the *Physical Activity Guidelines* complements the *Dietary Guidelines for Americans*, a joint effort of HHS and the U.S. Department of Agriculture (USDA). Together, the two documents provide guidance on the importance of being physically active and eating a healthy diet to promote good health and reduce the risk of chronic diseases.

The primary audiences for the *Physical Activity Guidelines* are policymakers and health professionals. These Guidelines are designed to provide information and guidance on the types and amounts of physical activity that provide substantial health benefits. This information may also be useful to interested members of the public. The main idea behind the Guidelines is that regular physical activity over months and years can produce long-term health benefits. Realizing these benefits requires physical activity each week.

Regular

physical activity can produce long-term health benefits.

The steps used to develop the *Physical Activity Guidelines for Americans* were similar to those used for the *Dietary Guidelines for Americans*. In 2007, HHS Secretary Mike Leavitt appointed an external scientific advisory committee, called the Physical Activity Guidelines Advisory Committee. The Advisory Committee conducted an extensive analysis of the scientific information on physical activity and health. The *Physical Activity Guidelines Advisory Committee Report, 2008* and meeting summaries are available at http://www.health.gov/PAGuidelines/.

HHS primarily used the Advisory Committee's report but also considered comments from the public and Government agencies when writing the Guidelines. The Guidelines will be widely promoted through various communications strategies, such as materials for the public, Web sites, and partnerships with organizations that promote physical activity.

The *Physical Activity Guidelines for Americans* describes the major research findings on the health benefits of physical activity:

- Regular physical activity reduces the risk of many adverse health outcomes.

- Some physical activity is better than none.

- For most health outcomes, additional benefits occur as the amount of physical activity increases through higher intensity, greater frequency, and/or longer duration.

- Most health benefits occur with at least 150 minutes (2 hours and 30 minutes) a week of moderate-intensity physical activity, such as brisk walking. Additional benefits occur with more physical activity.

- Both aerobic (endurance) and muscle-strengthening (resistance) physical activity are beneficial.

- Health benefits occur for children and adolescents, young and middle-aged adults, older adults, and those in every studied racial and ethnic group.

- The health benefits of physical activity occur for people with disabilities.

- The benefits of physical activity far outweigh the possibility of adverse outcomes.

The following are the key Guidelines included in the *Physical Activity Guidelines for Americans:*

Key Guidelines for Children and Adolescents

- Children and adolescents should do 60 minutes (1 hour) or more of physical activity daily.

  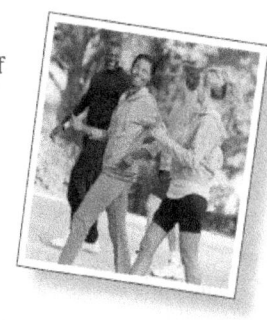

  - **Aerobic:** Most of the 60 or more minutes a day should be either moderate- or vigorous-intensity aerobic physical activity, and should include vigorous-intensity physical activity at least 3 days a week.

  - **Muscle-strengthening:** As part of their 60 or more minutes of daily physical activity, children and adolescents should include muscle-strengthening physical activity on at least 3 days of the week.

  - **Bone-strengthening:** As part of their 60 or more minutes of daily physical activity, children and adolescents should include bone-strengthening physical activity on at least 3 days of the week.

- It is important to encourage young people to participate in physical activities that are appropriate for their age, that are enjoyable, and that offer variety.

Key Guidelines for Adults

- All adults should avoid inactivity. Some physical activity is better than none, and adults who participate in any amount of physical activity gain some health benefits.

- For substantial health benefits, adults should do at least 150 minutes (2 hours and 30 minutes) a week of moderate-intensity, or 75 minutes (1 hour and 15 minutes) a week of vigorous-intensity aerobic physical activity, or an equivalent combination of moderate- and vigorous-intensity aerobic activity. Aerobic activity should be performed in episodes of at least 10 minutes, and preferably, it should be spread throughout the week.

- For additional and more extensive health benefits, adults should increase their aerobic physical activity to 300 minutes (5 hours) a week of moderate-intensity, or 150 minutes a week of vigorous-intensity aerobic physical activity, or an equivalent combination of moderate- and vigorous-intensity activity. Additional health benefits are gained by engaging in physical activity beyond this amount.

- Adults should also do muscle-strengthening activities that are moderate or high intensity and involve all major muscle groups on 2 or more days a week, as these activities provide additional health benefits.

Key Guidelines for Older Adults

The Key Guidelines for Adults also apply to older adults. In addition, the following Guidelines are just for older adults:

- When older adults cannot do 150 minutes of moderate-intensity aerobic activity a week because of chronic conditions, they should be as physically active as their abilities and conditions allow.

- Older adults should do exercises that maintain or improve balance if they are at risk of falling.

- Older adults should determine their level of effort for physical activity relative to their level of fitness.

- Older adults with chronic conditions should understand whether and how their conditions affect their ability to do regular physical activity safely.

Key Guidelines for Safe Physical Activity

To do physical activity safely and reduce the risk of injuries and other adverse events, people should:

- Understand the risks and yet be confident that physical activity is safe for almost everyone.

- Choose to do types of physical activity that are appropriate for their current fitness level and health goals, because some activities are safer than others.

- Increase physical activity gradually over time whenever more activity is necessary to meet guidelines or health goals. Inactive people should "start low and go slow" by gradually increasing how often and how long activities are done.

- Protect themselves by using appropriate gear and sports equipment, looking for safe environments, following rules and policies, and making sensible choices about when, where, and how to be active.

- Be under the care of a health-care provider if they have chronic conditions or symptoms. People with chronic conditions and symptoms should consult their health-care provider about the types and amounts of activity appropriate for them.

Key Guidelines for Women During Pregnancy and the Postpartum Period

- Healthy women who are not already highly active or doing vigorous-intensity activity should get at least 150 minutes of moderate-intensity aerobic activity a week during pregnancy and the postpartum period. Preferably, this activity should be spread throughout the week.

- Pregnant women who habitually engage in vigorous-intensity aerobic activity or who are highly active can continue physical activity during pregnancy and the postpartum period, provided that they remain healthy and discuss with their health-care provider how and when activity should be adjusted over time.

Key Guidelines for Adults With Disabilities

- Adults with disabilities, who are able to, should get at least 150 minutes a week of moderate-intensity, or 75 minutes a week of vigorous-intensity aerobic activity, or an equivalent combination of moderate- and vigorous-intensity aerobic activity. Aerobic activity should be performed in episodes of at least 10 minutes, and preferably, it should be spread throughout the week.

- Adults with disabilities, who are able to, should also do muscle-strengthening activities of moderate or high intensity that involve all major muscle groups on 2 or more days a week, as these activities provide additional health benefits.

- When adults with disabilities are not able to meet the Guidelines, they should engage in regular physical activity according to their abilities and should avoid inactivity.

- Adults with disabilities should consult their health-care provider about the amounts and types of physical activity that are appropriate for their abilities.

Key Messages for People With Chronic Medical Conditions

- Adults with chronic conditions obtain important health benefits from regular physical activity.

- When adults with chronic conditions do activity according to their abilities, physical activity is safe.

- Adults with chronic conditions should be under the care of a health-care provider. People with chronic conditions and symptoms should consult their health-care provider about the types and amounts of activity appropriate for them.

A Roadmap to the *2008 Physical Activity Guidelines for Americans*

- For an overview of the development of the *Physical Activity Guidelines for Americans* and important background information about physical activity, read **Chapter 1—Introducing the 2008 Physical Activity Guidelines for Americans.**

  NOTE

  The Guidelines assume that many readers will not read all the chapters, but will read only what is relevant to them. Important information may therefore be repeated in several chapters.

- To learn about the health benefits of physical activity, read **Chapter 2—Physical Activity Has Many Health Benefits.** This information may help motivate people to become regularly active.

- To understand how to do physical activity in a manner that meets the Guidelines:

  - For youth aged 6 to 17, including youth with disabilities, read **Chapter 3—Active Children and Adolescents.**

  - For adults aged 18 to 64, read **Chapter 4— Active Adults.**

  - For adults aged 65 and older, read **Chapter 5— Active Older Adults.** This chapter is also appropriate reading for adults younger than age 65 who have chronic conditions. The Guidelines for older adults are similar to those for other adults but add some specific considerations, such as guidelines for fall prevention.

  - For women who are pregnant or who have recently given birth (postpartum period), read the age-appropriate chapter and also the section on physical activity and pregnancy in **Chapter 6— Safe and Active** and **Chapter 7—Additional Considerations for Some Adults.**

  - For adults with disabilities, read **Chapter 4—Active Adults** and **Chapter 7—Additional Considerations for Some Adults.**

- To understand how to reduce the risks of activity-related injury, read **Chapter 6—Safe and Active.**

- Those interested in an overview of ways to help people participate regularly in physical activity should read **Chapter 8—Taking Action: Increasing Physical Activity Levels of Americans.**

- The **Glossary** contains definitions of key terms used in the Guidelines. Terms that are defined in the glossary are underlined the first time they are used.

- Additional information and resources relevant to the Guidelines are available in the **Appendices.**

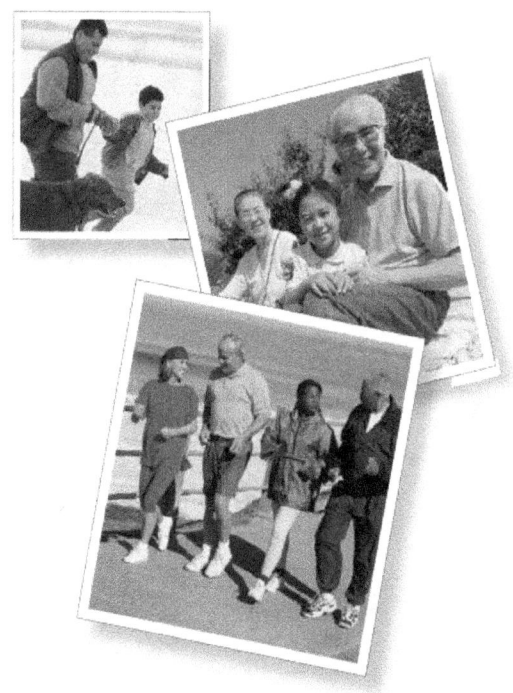

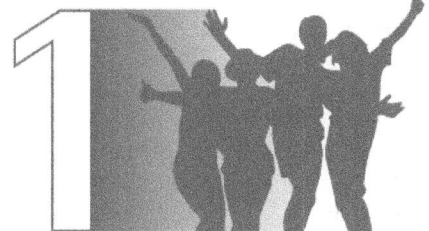

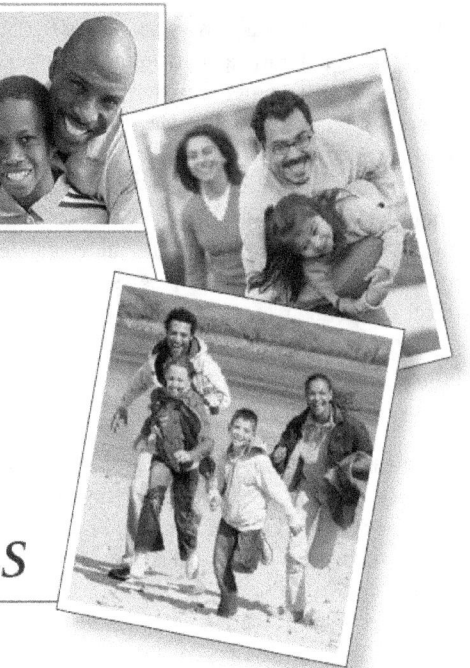

Introducing the *2008 Physical Activity Guidelines for Americans*

Being physically active is one of the most important steps that Americans of all ages can take to improve their <u>health</u>. This inaugural *Physical Activity Guidelines for Americans* provides science-based guidance to help Americans aged 6 and older improve their health through appropriate <u>physical activity</u>.

The U.S. Department of Health and Human Services (HHS) issues the *Physical Activity Guidelines for Americans*. The content of the *Physical Activity Guidelines* complements the *Dietary Guidelines for Americans*, a joint effort of HHS and the U.S. Department of Agriculture (USDA). Together, the two documents provide guidance on the importance of being physically active and eating a healthy diet to promote good health and reduce the risk of chronic diseases.

This chapter provides background information about the rationale and process for developing the Guidelines. It then discusses several issues that provide the framework for understanding the Guidelines. The chapter also explains how these Guidelines fit in with other published physical activity recommendations and how they should be used in practice.

Why and How the Guidelines Were Developed

The Rationale for Physical Activity Guidelines

We clearly know enough now to recommend that all Americans should engage in regular physical activity to improve overall health and to reduce risk of many health problems. Physical activity is a leading example of how lifestyle choices have a profound effect on health. The choices we make about other lifestyle factors, such as diet, smoking, and alcohol use, also have important and independent effects on our health.

The primary audiences for the *Physical Activity Guidelines for Americans* are policymakers and health professionals. The Guidelines are designed to provide information and guidance on the types and amounts of physical activity that provide substantial health benefits. This information may also be useful to interested members of the public. The main idea behind the Guidelines is that regular physical activity over months and years can produce long-term health benefits. Realizing these benefits requires physical activity each week.

These Guidelines are necessary because of the importance of physical activity to the health of Americans, whose current inactivity puts them at unnecessary risk. *Healthy People 2010* set objectives for increasing the level of physical activity in Americans over the decade from 2000 to 2010. Unfortunately, the latest information shows that inactivity among American adults and youth remains relatively high and that little progress has been made in meeting these objectives.

The Development of the Physical Activity Guidelines for Americans

Since 1995 the *Dietary Guidelines for Americans* has included advice on physical activity. However, with the development of a firm science base on the health benefits of physical activity, HHS began to consider whether separate physical activity guidelines were appropriate. With the help of the Institute of Medicine, HHS convened a workshop in October 2006 to address this question. The workshop's report, *Adequacy of Evidence for Physical Activity Guidelines Development* (http://www.nap.edu/catalog.php?record_id=11819), affirmed that advances in the science of physical activity and health justified the creation of separate physical activity guidelines.

The steps used to develop the *Physical Activity Guidelines for Americans* were similar to those used for the *Dietary Guidelines for Americans*. In 2007 HHS Secretary Mike Leavitt appointed an external scientific advisory committee called the Physical Activity Guidelines Advisory Committee. The Advisory Committee conducted an extensive analysis of the scientific information on physical activity and health. The *Physical Activity Guidelines Advisory Committee Report, 2008* and meeting summaries are available at http://www.health.gov/PAGuidelines/.

HHS primarily used the Advisory Committee's report but also considered comments from the public and Government agencies when writing the Guidelines. The Guidelines will be widely promoted through various communications strategies, such as materials for the public, Web sites, and partnerships with organizations that promote physical activity.

The Framework for the Physical Activity Guidelines for Americans

The Advisory Committee report provided the content and conceptual underpinning for the Guidelines. The main elements of this framework are described in the following sections.

Baseline Activity Versus Health-Enhancing Physical Activity

Physical activity has been defined as any bodily movement produced by the contraction of skeletal muscle that increases energy expenditure above a basal level. However, in this document, the term "physical activity" will generally refer to bodily movement that enhances health. Bodily movement can be divided into two categories:

- **Baseline activity** refers to the light-intensity activities of daily life, such as standing, walking slowly, and lifting lightweight objects. People vary in how much baseline activity they do. People who do only baseline activity are considered to be inactive. They may do very short episodes of moderate- or vigorous-intensity activity, such as climbing a few flights of stairs, but these episodes aren't long enough to count toward meeting the Guidelines. The Guidelines don't comment on how variations in types and amounts of baseline physical activity might affect health, as this was not addressed by the Advisory Committee report.

- **Health-enhancing physical activity** is activity that, when added to baseline activity, produces health benefits. In this document, the term "physical activity" generally refers to health-enhancing physical activity. Brisk walking, jumping rope, dancing, lifting weights, climbing on playground equipment at recess, and doing yoga are all examples of physical activity. Some people (such as postal carriers or carpenters on construction sites) may get enough physical activity on the job to meet the Guidelines.

We don't understand enough about whether doing more baseline activity results in health benefits. Even so, efforts to promote baseline activities are justifiable. After all, baseline activities are normal

In this document,

the term "physical activity" will generally refer to bodily movement that enhances health.

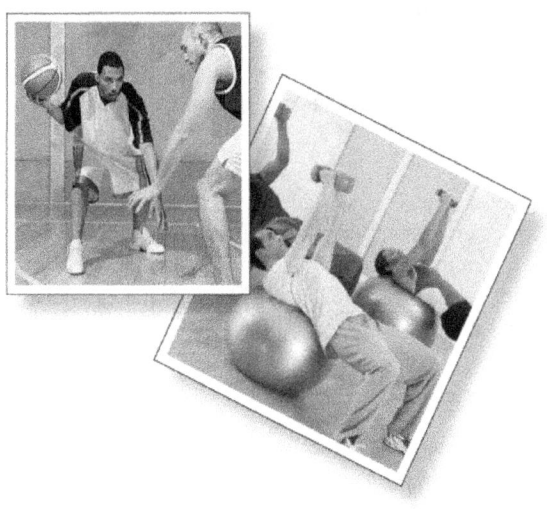

lifestyle activities. Encouraging Americans to increase their baseline activity is sensible for several reasons:

- Increasing baseline activity burns calories, which can help in maintaining a healthy body weight.

- Some baseline activities are weight-bearing and may improve bone health.

- There are reasons other than health to encourage more baseline activity. For example, walking short distances instead of driving can help reduce traffic congestion and the resulting air pollution.

- Encouraging baseline activities helps build a culture where physical activity in general is the social norm.

- Short episodes of activity are appropriate for people who were inactive and have started to gradually increase their level of activity, and for older adults whose activity may be limited by chronic conditions.

The availability of infrastructure to support short episodes of activity is therefore important. For example, people should have the option of using sidewalks and paths to walk between buildings at a worksite, rather than having to drive. People should also have the option of taking the stairs instead of using an elevator.

Health Benefits Versus Other Reasons To Be Physically Active

Although the Guidelines focus on the health benefits of physical activity, these benefits are not the only reason why people are active. Physical activity gives people a chance to have fun, be with friends and family, enjoy the outdoors, improve their personal appearance, and improve their fitness so that they can participate in more intensive physical activity or sporting events. Some people are active because they feel it gives them certain health benefits (such as feeling more energetic) that aren't yet conclusively proven for the general population.

The Guidelines encourage people to be physically active for any and all reasons that are meaningful for them. Nothing in the Guidelines is intended to mean that health benefits are the only reason to do physical activity.

Focus on Disease Prevention

The Guidelines focus on preventive effects of physical activity, which include lowering the risk of developing chronic diseases such as heart disease and type 2 diabetes.

Physical activity also has beneficial therapeutic effects and is commonly recommended as part of the treatment for medical conditions. The Advisory Committee report did not review the therapeutic effects of activity, and the Guidelines do not discuss the use of physical activity as medical treatment.

Health-Related Versus Performance-Related Fitness

The Guidelines focus on reducing the risk of chronic disease and promoting health-related fitness, particularly cardiovascular and muscular fitness. People can gain this kind of fitness by doing the amount and types of activities recommended in the Guidelines.

The Guidelines do not address the types and amounts of activity necessary to improve _performance-related fitness_. Athletes need this kind of fitness when they compete. Medical screening issues for competitive athletes also are outside the scope of the Guidelines.

People who are interested in training programs to increase performance-related fitness should seek advice from other sources. Generally, these people do much more activity than required to meet the Guidelines.

Lifespan Approach

The best way to be physically active is to be active for life. Therefore, the Guidelines take a lifespan approach and provide recommendations for three age groups: Children and Adolescents, Adults, and Older Adults.

The _Physical Activity Guidelines_ are for Americans aged 6 and older. The Advisory Committee report did not review evidence for children younger than age 6. Physical activity in infants and young children is, of course, necessary for healthy growth and development. Children younger than 6 should be physically active in ways appropriate for their age and stage of development.

Individualized Health Goals

The Guidelines generally explain the amounts and types of physical activity needed for health benefits.

Within these overall parameters, individuals have many choices about appropriate types and amounts of activity.

To make these choices, American adults need to set personal goals for physical activity. Setting these goals involves questions like, "How physically fit do I want to be?" "How important is it to me to reduce my risk of heart disease and diabetes?" "How important is it to me to reduce my risk of falls and hip fracture?" "How much weight do I want to lose and keep off?"

People can meet the Guidelines and their own personal goals through different amounts and types of activity. Written materials, health-care providers, and fitness professionals can provide useful information and help people set and carry out specific goals.

Four Levels of Physical Activity

The Advisory Committee report provides the basis for dividing the amount of <u>aerobic physical activity</u> an adult gets every week into four categories: inactive, low, medium, and high (see table below). This classification is useful because these categories provide a rule of thumb of how total amount of physical activity is related to health benefits. Low amounts of activity provide some benefits; medium amounts provide substantial benefits; and high amounts provide even greater benefits.

Classification of Total Weekly Amounts of Aerobic Physical Activity Into Four Categories

Levels of Physical Activity	Range of Moderate-Intensity Minutes a Week	Summary of Overall Health Benefits	Comment
Inactive	No activity beyond baseline	None	Being inactive is unhealthy.
Low	Activity beyond baseline but fewer than 150 minutes a week	Some	Low levels of activity are clearly preferable to an inactive lifestyle.
Medium	150 minutes to 300 minutes a week	Substantial	Activity at the high end of this range has additional and more extensive health benefits than activity at the low end.
High	More than 300 minutes a week	Additional	Current science does not allow researchers to identify an upper limit of activity above which there are no additional health benefits.

Action is needed

at the individual, community, and societal levels to help Americans become physically active.

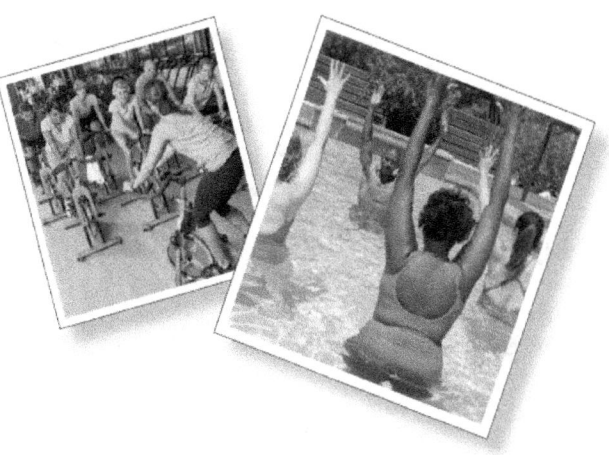

- **Inactive** is no activity beyond baseline activities of daily living.

- **Low activity** is activity beyond baseline but fewer than 150 minutes (2 hours and 30 minutes) of <u>moderate-intensity physical activity</u> a week or the equivalent amount (75 minutes, or 1 hour and 15 minutes) of vigorous-intensity activity.

- **Medium activity** is 150 minutes to 300 (5 hours) minutes of moderate-intensity activity a week (or 75 to 150 minutes of <u>vigorous-intensity physical activity</u> a week). In scientific terms, this range is approximately equivalent to 500 to 1,000 metabolic equivalent (<u>MET</u>) minutes a week.

> **For More Information**
>
> Appendix 1 provides a detailed explanation of MET-minutes, a unit useful for describing the energy expenditure of a specific physical activity.

- **High activity** is more than the equivalent of 300 minutes of moderate-intensity physical activity a week.

Relationship to Previous Public Health Recommendations

In 1995 the Centers for Disease Control and Prevention (CDC) and the American College of Sports Medicine (ACSM) published physical activity recommendations for public health. The report stated that adults should <u>accumulate</u> at least 30 minutes a day of moderate-intensity physical activity on most, preferably all, days per week. In 1996 *Physical Activity and Health: A Report of the Surgeon General* supported this same recommendation.

In order to track the percentage of adults who meet this guideline, CDC specified that "most" days per week was 5 days. Since 1995 the common recommendation has been that adults obtain at least 30 minutes of

moderate-intensity physical activity on 5 or more days a week, for a total of at least 150 minutes a week.

The *Physical Activity Guidelines for Americans* affirms that it is acceptable to follow the CDC/ACSM recommendation and similar recommendations. However, according to the Advisory Committee report, the CDC/ACSM guideline was too specific. In other words, existing scientific evidence does not allow researchers to say, for example, whether the health benefits of 30 minutes on 5 days a week are any different from the health benefits of 50 minutes on 3 days a week. As a result, the new Guidelines allow a person to accumulate 150 minutes a week in various ways.

Putting the Guidelines Into Practice

Although the Advisory Committee did not review strategies to promote physical activity, action is needed at the individual, community, and societal levels to help Americans become physically active. Publications such as the *Guide to Community Preventive Services* (http://www.thecommunityguide.org/pa/) and the recommendations of the U.S. Preventive Services Task Force (http://www.ahrq.gov/clinic/cps3dix.htm) summarize evidence-based strategies for promoting physical activity on the community level and through primary health care. Accordingly, the final chapter of the *Physical Activity Guidelines for Americans* provides only a brief discussion on promoting physical activity, and indicates how to link the Guidelines to action strategies.

Assessing Whether Physical Activity Programs Are Consistent With the Guidelines

Programs that provide opportunities for physical activity, such as classes or community activities, can help people meet the Guidelines. These programs do not have to provide all, or even most, of the recommended weekly activity. For example, a mall walking program for older adults may meet only once a week yet provide useful amounts of activity, as long as people get the rest of their weekly recommended activity on other days.

Programs that are consistent with the Guidelines:

- Provide advice and education consistent with the Guidelines;

- Add episodes of activity that count toward meeting the Guidelines; and

- May also include activities, such as stretching or warming up and cooling down, whose health benefits are not yet proven but that are often used in effective physical activity programs.

The Importance of Understandable Guidelines

HHS has tried to keep the *Physical Activity Guidelines* straightforward and clear, while remaining consistent with complex scientific information. In each chapter the key Guidelines are set apart from the text, in order to identify the most important information to communicate to the public. The messages contained in these Guidelines should be disseminated to the general public and to anyone involved in promoting physical activity.

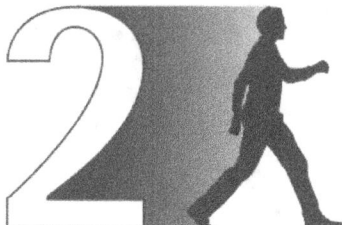

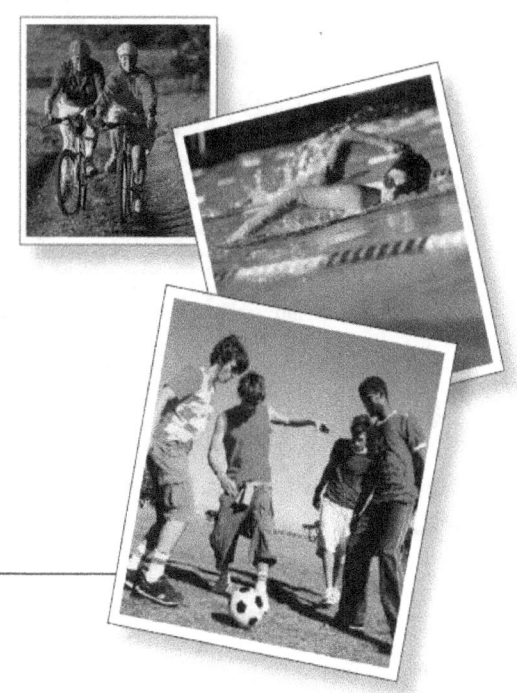

Physical Activity Has
Many Health Benefits

All Americans should be regularly physically active to improve overall health and fitness and to prevent many adverse health outcomes. The benefits of physical activity occur in generally healthy people, in people at risk of developing chronic diseases, and in people with current chronic conditions or disabilities. This chapter gives an overview of research findings on physical activity and health. The box on page 8 provides a summary of these benefits.

Physical activity affects many health conditions, and the specific amounts and types of activity that benefit each condition vary. In developing public health guidelines, the challenge is to integrate scientific information across all health benefits and identify a critical range of physical activity that appears to have an effect across the health benefits. One consistent finding from research studies is that once the health benefits from physical activity begin to accrue, additional amounts of activity provide additional benefits.

Although some health benefits seem to begin with as little as 60 minutes (1 hour) a week, research shows that a total amount of 150 minutes (2 hours and 30 minutes) a week of moderate-intensity aerobic activity, such as

brisk walking, consistently reduces the risk of many chronic diseases and other adverse health outcomes.

Examining the Relationship Between Physical Activity and Health

In many studies covering a wide range of issues, researchers have focused on <u>exercise</u>, as well as on the more broadly defined concept of physical activity. Exercise is a form of physical activity that is planned, structured, repetitive, and performed with the goal of improving health or fitness. So, although all exercise is physical activity, not all physical activity is exercise.

Studies have examined the role of physical activity in many groups—men and women, children, teens, adults, older adults, people with disabilities, and women during pregnancy and the postpartum period. These studies have focused on the role that physical activity plays in many health outcomes, including:

- Premature (early) death;
- Diseases such as coronary heart disease, stroke, some cancers, type 2 diabetes, osteoporosis, and depression;

The Health Benefits of Physical Activity—Major Research Findings

- Regular physical activity reduces the risk of many adverse health outcomes.

- Some physical activity is better than none.

- For most health outcomes, additional benefits occur as the amount of physical activity increases through higher intensity, greater frequency, and/or longer duration.

- Most health benefits occur with at least 150 minutes a week of moderate-intensity physical activity, such as brisk walking. Additional benefits occur with more physical activity.

- Both aerobic (endurance) and muscle-strengthening (resistance) physical activity are beneficial.

- Health benefits occur for children and adolescents, young and middle-aged adults, older adults, and those in every studied racial and ethnic group.

- The health benefits of physical activity occur for people with disabilities.

- The benefits of physical activity far outweigh the possibility of adverse outcomes.

- Risk factors for disease, such as high blood pressure and high blood cholesterol;

- Physical fitness, such as aerobic capacity, and muscle strength and endurance;

- Functional capacity (the ability to engage in activities needed for daily living);

- Mental health, such as depression and cognitive function; and

- Injuries or sudden heart attacks.

These studies have also prompted questions as to what type and how much physical activity is needed for various health benefits. To answer this question, investigators have studied three main kinds of physical activity: aerobic, muscle-strengthening, and bone-strengthening. Investigators have also studied balance and flexibility activities. These latter two activities are addressed in Chapters 4, 5, and 6.

Aerobic Activity

In this kind of physical activity (also called an endurance activity or cardio activity), the body's large muscles move in a rhythmic manner for a sustained period of time. Brisk walking, running, bicycling, jumping rope, and swimming are all examples.

Aerobic activity causes a person's heart to beat faster than usual.

Aerobic physical activity has three components:

- **Intensity,** or how hard a person works to do the activity. The intensities most often examined are moderate intensity (equivalent in effort to brisk walking) and vigorous intensity (equivalent in effort to running or jogging);

- **Frequency,** or how often a person does aerobic activity; and

- **Duration,** or how long a person does an activity in any one session.

Although these components make up a physical activity profile, research has shown that the total amount of physical activity (minutes of moderate-intensity physical activity, for example) is more important for achieving health benefits than is any one component (frequency, intensity, or duration).

Muscle-Strengthening Activity

This kind of activity, which includes resistance training and lifting weights, causes the body's muscles to work or hold against an applied force or weight. These activities often involve relatively heavy objects, such as weights, which are lifted multiple times to train various muscle groups. Muscle-strengthening activity can also be done by using elastic bands or body weight for resistance (climbing a tree or doing push-ups, for example).

Muscle-strengthening activity also has three components:

- **Intensity,** or how much weight or force is used relative to how much a person is able to lift;

- **Frequency,** or how often a person does muscle-strengthening activity; and

- **Repetitions,** or how many times a person lifts a weight (analogous to duration for aerobic activity).

The effects of muscle-strengthening activity are limited to the muscles doing the work. It's important to work all the major muscle groups of the body: the legs, hips, back, abdomen, chest, shoulders, and arms.

Bone-Strengthening Activity

This kind of activity (sometimes called weight-bearing or weight-loading activity) produces a force on the bones that promotes bone growth and strength. This force is commonly produced by impact with the ground. Examples of bone-strengthening activity include jumping jacks, running, brisk walking, and weight-lifting exercises. As these examples illustrate, bone-strengthening activities can also be aerobic and muscle strengthening.

The Health Benefits of Physical Activity

Studies clearly demonstrate that participating in regular physical activity provides many health benefits. These benefits are summarized in the accompanying table. Many conditions affected by physical activity occur with increasing age, such as heart disease and cancer. Reducing risk of these conditions may require years of participation in regular physical activity. However, other benefits, such as increased cardiorespiratory fitness, increased muscular strength, and decreased depressive symptoms and blood pressure, require only a few weeks or months of participation in physical activity.

Health Benefits Associated With Regular Physical Activity

Children and Adolescents

Strong evidence

- Improved cardiorespiratory and muscular fitness
- Improved bone health
- Improved cardiovascular and metabolic health biomarkers
- Favorable body composition

Moderate evidence

- Reduced symptoms of depression

Adults and Older Adults

Strong evidence

- Lower risk of early death
- Lower risk of coronary heart disease
- Lower risk of stroke
- Lower risk of high blood pressure
- Lower risk of adverse blood lipid profile
- Lower risk of type 2 diabetes
- Lower risk of metabolic syndrome
- Lower risk of colon cancer
- Lower risk of breast cancer
- Prevention of weight gain
- Weight loss, particularly when combined with reduced calorie intake
- Improved cardiorespiratory and muscular fitness
- Prevention of falls
- Reduced depression
- Better cognitive function (for older adults)

Moderate to strong evidence

- Better functional health (for older adults)
- Reduced abdominal obesity

Moderate evidence

- Lower risk of hip fracture
- Lower risk of lung cancer
- Lower risk of endometrial cancer
- Weight maintenance after weight loss
- Increased bone density
- Improved sleep quality

Note: The Advisory Committee rated the evidence of health benefits of physical activity as strong, moderate, or weak. To do so, the Committee considered the type, number, and quality of studies available, as well as consistency of findings across studies that addressed each outcome. The Committee also considered evidence for causality and dose response in assigning the strength-of-evidence rating.

The Beneficial Effects of Increasing Physical Activity: It's About Overload, Progression, and Specificity

<u>Overload</u> is the physical stress placed on the body when physical activity is greater in amount or intensity than usual. The body's structures and functions respond and <u>adapt</u> to these stresses. For example, aerobic physical activity places a stress on the cardiorespiratory system and muscles, requiring the lungs to move more air and the heart to pump more blood and deliver it to the working muscles. This increase in demand increases the efficiency and capacity of the lungs, heart, circulatory system, and exercising muscles. In the same way, muscle-strengthening and bone-strengthening activities overload muscles and bones, making them stronger.

<u>Progression</u> is closely tied to overload. Once a person reaches a certain fitness level, he or she progresses to higher levels of physical activity by continued overload and adaptation. Small, progressive changes in overload help the body adapt to the additional stresses while minimizing the risk of injury.

<u>Specificity</u> means that the benefits of physical activity are specific to the body systems that are doing the work. For example, aerobic physical activity largely benefits the body's cardiovascular system.

The health benefits of physical activity are seen in children and adolescents, young and middle-aged adults, older adults, women and men, people of different races and ethnicities, and people with disabilities and chronic conditions. The health benefits of physical activity are generally independent of body weight. Adults of all sizes and shapes gain health and fitness benefits by being habitually physically active. The benefits of physical activity also outweigh the risk of injury and sudden heart attacks, two concerns that prevent many people from becoming physically active.

The following sections provide more detail on what is known from research studies about the specific health benefits of physical activity and how much physical activity is needed to get the health benefits.

Premature Death

Strong scientific evidence shows that physical activity reduces the risk of premature death (dying earlier than the average age of death for a specific population group) from the leading causes of death, such as heart disease and some cancers, as well as from other causes of death. This effect is remarkable in two ways:

- First, only a few lifestyle choices have as large an effect on mortality as physical activity. It has been estimated that people who are physically active for approximately 7 hours a week have a 40 percent lower risk of dying early than those who are active for less than 30 minutes a week.

- Second, it is not necessary to do high amounts of activity or vigorous-intensity activity to reduce the risk of premature death. Studies show substantially lower risk when people do 150 minutes of at least moderate-intensity aerobic physical activity a week.

Research clearly demonstrates the importance of avoiding inactivity. Even low amounts of physical activity reduce the risk of dying prematurely. As the figure on page 11 shows, the most dramatic difference in risk is seen between those who are inactive (30 minutes a week) and those with low levels of activity (90 minutes or 1 hour and 30 minutes a week). The <u>relative risk</u> of dying prematurely continues to be lower with higher levels of reported moderate- or vigorous-intensity leisure-time physical activity.

All adults can gain this health benefit of physical activity. Age, race, and ethnicity do not matter. Men and women younger than 65 years as well as older adults have lower rates of early death when they are physically active than when they are inactive. Physically active people of all body weights (normal weight, overweight, obese) also have lower rates of early death than do inactive people.

The Risk of Dying Prematurely Declines as People Become Physically Active

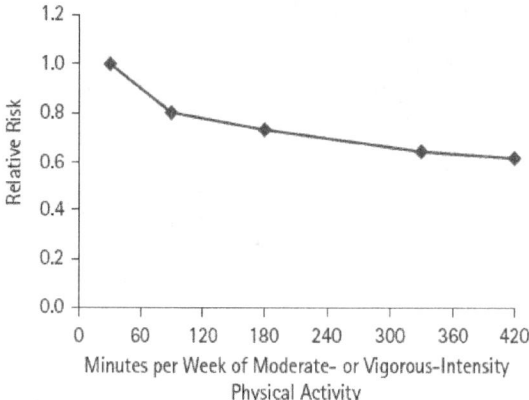

Relative Risk (y-axis)

Minutes per Week of Moderate- or Vigorous-Intensity Physical Activity (x-axis)

Cardiorespiratory Health

The benefits of physical activity on cardiorespiratory health are some of the most extensively documented of all the health benefits. Cardiorespiratory health involves the health of the heart, lungs, and blood vessels.

Heart diseases and stroke are two of the leading causes of death in the United States. Risk factors that increase the likelihood of cardiovascular diseases include smoking, high blood pressure (called hypertension), type 2 diabetes, and high levels of certain blood lipids (such as low-density lipoprotein, or LDL, cholesterol). Low cardiorespiratory fitness also is a risk factor for heart disease.

People who do moderate- or vigorous-intensity aerobic physical activity have a significantly lower risk of cardiovascular disease than do inactive people. Regularly active adults have lower rates of heart disease and stroke, and have lower blood pressure, better blood lipid profiles, and fitness. Significant reductions in risk of cardiovascular disease occur at activity levels equivalent to 150 minutes a week of moderate-intensity physical activity. Even greater benefits are seen with 200 minutes (3 hours and 20 minutes) a week. The evidence is strong that greater amounts of physical activity result in even further reductions in the risk of cardiovascular disease.

Everyone can gain the cardiovascular health benefits of physical activity. The amount of physical activity

that provides favorable cardiorespiratory health and fitness outcomes is similar for adults of various ages, including older people, as well as for adults of various races and ethnicities. Aerobic exercise also improves cardiorespiratory fitness in individuals with some disabilities, including people who have lost the use of one or both legs and those with multiple sclerosis, stroke, spinal cord injury, and cognitive disabilities.

Moderate-intensity physical activity is safe for generally healthy women during pregnancy. It increases cardiorespiratory fitness without increasing the risk of early pregnancy loss, preterm delivery, or low birth weight. Physical activity during the postpartum period also improves cardiorespiratory fitness.

Metabolic Health

Regular physical activity strongly reduces the risk of developing type 2 diabetes as well as the metabolic syndrome. The metabolic syndrome is defined as a condition in which people have some combination of high blood pressure, a large waistline (abdominal obesity), an adverse blood lipid profile (low levels of high-density lipoprotein [HDL] cholesterol, raised triglycerides), and impaired glucose tolerance.

People who regularly engage in at least moderate-intensity aerobic activity have a significantly lower risk of developing type 2 diabetes than do inactive people. Although some experts debate the usefulness of defining the metabolic syndrome, good evidence exists that physical activity reduces the risk of having this condition, as defined in various ways. Lower rates of these conditions are seen with 120 to 150 minutes (2 hours to 2 hours and 30 minutes) a week of at least moderate-intensity aerobic activity. As with cardiovascular health, additional levels of physical activity seem to lower risk even further. In addition, physical activity helps control blood glucose levels in persons who already have type 2 diabetes.

Physical activity also improves metabolic health in youth. Studies find this effect when young people participate in at least 3 days of vigorous aerobic activity a week. More physical activity is associated with improved metabolic health, but research has yet to determine the exact amount of improvement.

Obesity and Energy Balance

Overweight and obesity occur when fewer calories are expended, including calories burned through physical activity, than are taken in through food and beverages. Physical activity and caloric intake both must be considered when trying to control body weight. Because of this role in energy balance, physical activity is a critical factor in determining whether a person can maintain a healthy body weight, lose excess body weight, or maintain successful weight loss. People vary a great deal in how much physical activity they need to achieve and maintain a healthy weight. Some need more physical activity than others to maintain a healthy body weight, to lose weight, or to keep weight off once it has been lost.

Strong scientific evidence shows that physical activity helps people maintain a stable weight over time. However, the optimal amount of physical activity needed to maintain weight is unclear. People vary greatly in how much physical activity results in weight stability. Many people need more than the equivalent of 150 minutes of moderate-intensity activity a week to maintain their weight.

Over short periods of time, such as a year, research shows that it is possible to achieve weight stability by doing the equivalent of 150 to 300 minutes (5 hours) a week of moderate-intensity walking at about a 4 mile-an-hour pace. Muscle-strengthening activities may help promote weight maintenance, although not to the same degree as aerobic activity.

People who want to lose a substantial (more than 5 percent of body weight) amount of weight and people who are trying to keep a significant amount of weight off once it has been lost need a high amount of physical activity unless they also reduce their caloric intake. Many people need to do more than 300 minutes of moderate-intensity activity a week to meet weight-control goals.

Regular physical activity also helps control the percentage of body fat in children and adolescents. Exercise training studies with overweight and obese youth have shown that they can reduce their body fatness by participating in physical activity that is at

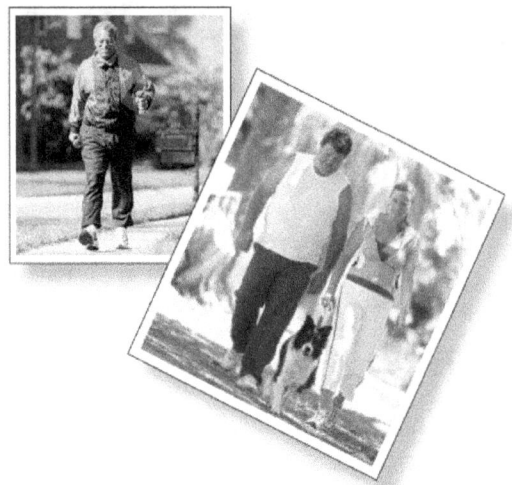

least moderate intensity on 3 to 5 days a week, for 30 to 60 minutes each time.

Musculoskeletal Health

Bones, muscles, and joints support the body and help it move. Healthy bones, joints, and muscles are critical to the ability to do daily activities without physical limitations.

Preserving bone, joint, and muscle health is essential with increasing age. Studies show that the frequent decline in bone density that happens during aging can be slowed with regular physical activity. These effects are seen in people who participate in aerobic, muscle-strengthening, and bone-strengthening physical activity programs of moderate or vigorous intensity. The range of total physical activity for these benefits varies widely. Important changes seem to begin at 90 minutes a week and continue up to 300 minutes a week.

Hip fracture is a serious health condition that can have life-changing negative effects for many older people. Physically active people, especially women, appear to have a lower risk of hip fracture than do inactive people. Research studies on physical activity to prevent hip fracture show that participating in 120 to 300 minutes a week of physical activity that is of at least moderate intensity is associated with a reduced risk. It is unclear, however, whether activity also lowers risk of fractures of the spine or other important areas of the skeleton.

The bottom line

is that the health benefits of physical activity far outweigh the risks of adverse events for almost everyone.

Building strong, healthy bones is also important for children and adolescents. Along with having a healthy diet that includes adequate calcium and vitamin D, physical activity is critical for bone development in children and adolescents. Bone-strengthening physical activity done 3 or more days a week increases bone-mineral content and bone density in youth.

Regular physical activity also helps people with arthritis or other rheumatic conditions affecting the joints. Participation in 130 to 150 minutes (2 hours and 10 minutes to 2 hours and 30 minutes) a week of moderate-intensity, low-impact physical activity improves pain management, function, and quality of life. Researchers don't yet know whether participation in physical activity, particularly at low to moderate intensity, reduces the risk of osteoarthritis. Very high levels of physical activity, however, may have extra risks. People who participate in very high levels of physical activity, such as elite or professional athletes, have a higher risk of hip and knee osteoarthritis, mostly due to the risk of injury involved in competing in some sports.

Progressive muscle-strengthening activities increase or preserve muscle mass, strength, and power. Higher amounts (through greater frequency or higher weights) improve muscle function to a greater degree. Improvements occur in younger and older adults. Resistance exercises also improve muscular strength in persons with such conditions as stroke, multiple sclerosis, cerebral palsy, spinal cord injury, and cognitive disability. Though it doesn't increase muscle mass in the same way that muscle-strengthening activities do, aerobic activity may also help slow the loss of muscle with aging.

Functional Ability and Fall Prevention

Functional ability is the capacity of a person to perform tasks or behaviors that enable him or her to carry out everyday activities, such as climbing stairs or walking on a sidewalk. Functional ability is key to a person's ability to fulfill basic life roles, such as personal care, grocery shopping, or playing with the grandchildren. Loss of functional ability is referred to as functional limitation.

Middle-aged and older adults who are physically active have lower risk of functional limitations than do inactive adults. It appears that greater physical activity levels can further reduce risk of functional limitations.

Older adults who already have functional limitations also benefit from regular physical activity. Typically, studies of physical activity in adults with functional limitations tested a combination of aerobic and muscle-strengthening activities, making it difficult to assess the relative importance of each type of activity. However, both types of activity appear to provide benefit.

In older adults at risk of falls, strong evidence shows that regular physical activity is safe and reduces this risk. Reduction in falls is seen for participants in programs that include balance and moderate-intensity muscle-strengthening activities for 90 minutes a week plus moderate-intensity walking for about an hour a week. It's not known whether different combinations of type, amount, or frequency of activity can reduce falls to a greater degree. Tai chi exercises also may help prevent falls.

Cancer

Physically active people have a significantly lower risk of colon cancer than do inactive people, and physically active women have a significantly lower risk of breast cancer. Research shows that a wide range of moderate-intensity physical activity—between 210 and 420 minutes a week (3 hours and 30 minutes to 7 hours)—is needed to significantly reduce the risk of colon and breast cancer; currently, 150 minutes a week does not appear to provide a major benefit. It also appears that greater amounts of physical activity lower risks of these cancers even further, although exactly how much lower is not clear.

Although not definitive, some research suggests that the risk of endometrial cancer in women and lung cancers in men and women also may be lower among those who are regularly active compared to those who are inactive.

Finally, cancer survivors have a better quality of life and improved physical fitness if they are physically active, compared to survivors who are inactive.

Mental Health

Physically active adults have lower risk of depression and cognitive decline (declines with aging in thinking, learning, and judgment skills). Physical activity also may improve the quality of sleep. Whether physical activity reduces distress or anxiety is currently unclear.

Mental health benefits have been found in people who do aerobic or a combination of aerobic and muscle-strengthening activities 3 to 5 days a week for 30 to 60 minutes at a time. Some research has shown that even lower levels of physical activity also may provide some benefits.

Regular physical activity appears to reduce symptoms of anxiety and depression for children and adolescents. Whether physical activity improves self-esteem is not clear.

Adverse Events

Some people hesitate to become active or increase their level of physical activity because they fear getting injured or having a heart attack. Studies of generally healthy people clearly show that moderate-intensity physical activity, such as brisk walking, has a low risk of such adverse events.

The risk of musculoskeletal injury increases with the total amount of physical activity. For example, a person who regularly runs 40 miles a week has a higher risk of injury than a person who runs 10 miles each week. However, people who are physically active may

have fewer injuries from other causes, such as motor vehicle collisions or work-related injuries. Depending on the type and amount of activity that physically active people do, their overall injury rate may be lower than the overall injury rate for inactive people.

Participation in contact or collision sports, such as soccer or football, has a higher risk of injury than participation in non-contact physical activity, such as swimming or walking. However, when performing the same activity, people who are less fit are more likely to be injured than people who are fitter.

Cardiac events, such as a heart attack or sudden death during physical activity, are rare. However, the risk of such cardiac events does increase when a person suddenly becomes much more active than usual. The greatest risk occurs when an adult who is usually inactive engages in vigorous-intensity activity (such as shoveling snow). People who are regularly physically active have the lowest risk of cardiac events both while being active and overall.

The bottom line is that the health benefits of physical activity far outweigh the risks of adverse events for almost everyone.

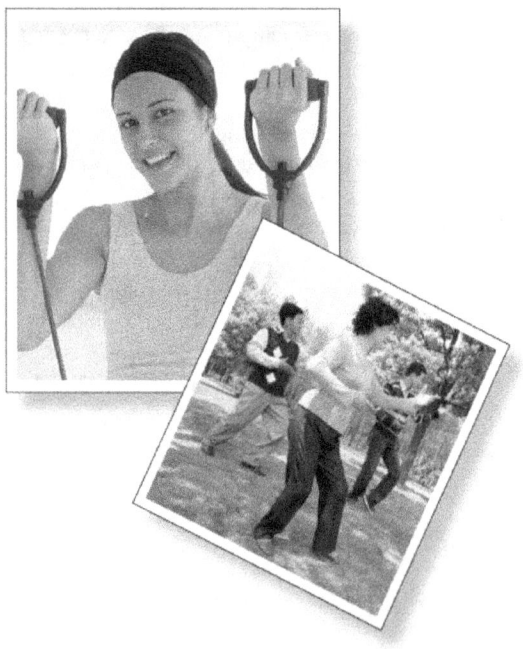

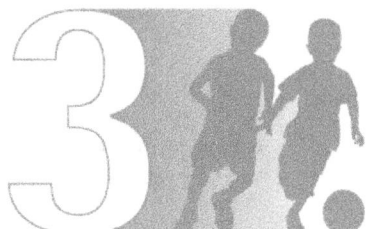

Active Children and Adolescents

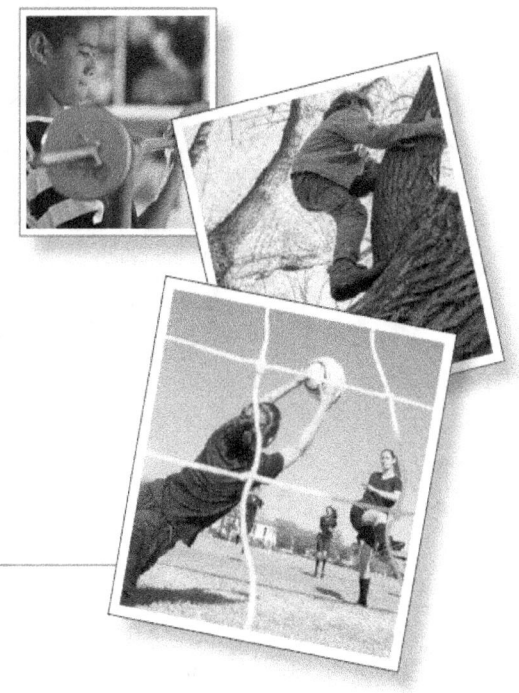

Regular physical activity in children and adolescents promotes health and fitness. Compared to those who are inactive, physically active youth have higher levels of cardiorespiratory fitness and stronger muscles. They also typically have lower body fatness. Their bones are stronger, and they may have reduced symptoms of anxiety and depression.

Youth who are regularly active also have a better chance of a healthy adulthood. Children and adolescents don't usually develop chronic diseases, such as heart disease, hypertension, type 2 diabetes, or osteoporosis. However, risk factors for these diseases can begin to develop early in life. Regular physical activity makes it less likely that these risk factors will develop and more likely that children will remain healthy as adults.

Youth can achieve substantial health benefits by doing moderate- and vigorous-intensity physical activity for periods of time that add up to 60 minutes (1 hour) or more each day. This activity should include aerobic activity as well as age-appropriate muscle- and bone-strengthening activities. Although current science is not complete, it appears that, as with adults, the total amount of physical activity is more important for achieving health benefits than is any one component (frequency, intensity, or duration) or specific mix of activities (aerobic, muscle-strengthening, bone-strengthening). Even so, bone-strengthening activities remain especially important for children and young adolescents because the greatest gains in bone mass occur during the years just before and during puberty. In addition, the majority of peak bone mass is obtained by the end of adolescence.

This chapter provides physical activity guidance for children and adolescents aged 6 to 17, and focuses on physical activity beyond baseline activity.

Parents and other adults who work with or care for youth should be familiar with the Guidelines in this chapter. These adults should be aware that, as children become adolescents, they typically reduce their physical activity. Adults play an important role in providing age-appropriate opportunities for physical activity. In doing so, they help lay an important foundation for life-long, health-promoting physical activity. Adults need to encourage active play in children and encourage sustained and structured activity as children grow older.

Explaining the Guidelines

Types of Activity

The Guidelines for children and adolescents focus on three types of activity: aerobic, muscle-strengthening, and bone-strengthening. Each type has important health benefits.

- **Aerobic activities** are those in which young people rhythmically move their large muscles. Running, hopping, skipping, jumping rope, swimming, dancing, and bicycling are all examples of aerobic activities. Aerobic activities increase cardiorespiratory fitness. Children often do activities in short bursts, which may not technically be aerobic activities. However, this document will also use the term aerobic to refer to these brief activities.

- **Muscle-strengthening activities** make muscles do more work than usual during activities of daily life. This is called "overload," and it strengthens the muscles. Muscle-strengthening activities can be unstructured and part of play, such as playing on playground equipment, climbing trees, and playing tug-of-war. Or these activities can be structured, such as lifting weights or working with resistance bands.

> **For More Information**
>
> See Chapter 2—Physical Activity Has Many Health Benefits, for more on overload and progression.

- **Bone-strengthening activities** produce a force on the bones that promotes bone growth and strength. This force is commonly produced by impact with the ground. Running, jumping rope, basketball, tennis, and hopscotch are all examples of bone-strengthening activities. As these examples illustrate, bone-strengthening activities can also be aerobic and muscle-strengthening.

How Age Influences Physical Activity in Children and Adolescents

Children and adolescents should meet the Guidelines by doing activity that is appropriate for their age. Their natural patterns of movement differ from those of adults. For example, children are naturally active in an intermittent way, particularly when they do unstructured active play. During recess and in their free play and games, children use basic aerobic and bone-strengthening activities, such as running, hopping, skipping, and jumping, to develop movement patterns and skills. They alternate brief periods of moderate- and vigorous-intensity activity with brief periods of rest. Any episode of moderate- or vigorous-intensity physical activity, however brief, counts toward the Guidelines.

Children also commonly increase muscle strength through unstructured activities that involve lifting or moving their body weight or working against resistance. Children don't usually do or need formal muscle-strengthening programs, such as lifting weights.

Regular physical

activity in children and adolescents promotes a healthy body weight and body composition.

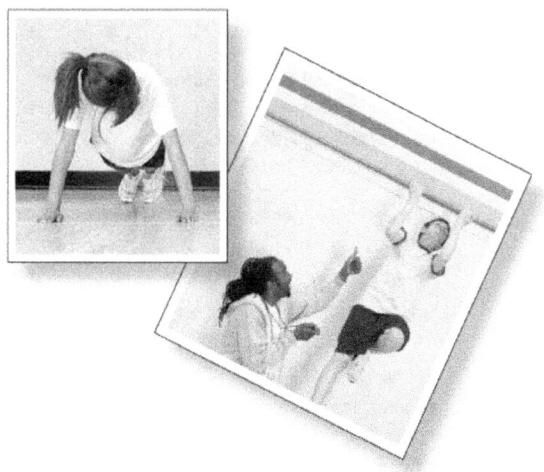

As children grow into adolescents, their patterns of physical activity change. They are able to play organized games and sports and are able to sustain longer periods of activity. But they still commonly do intermittent activity, and no period of moderate- or vigorous-intensity activity is too short to count toward the Guidelines.

Adolescents may meet the Guidelines by doing free play, structured programs, or both. Structured exercise programs can include aerobic activities, such as playing a sport, and muscle-strengthening activities, such as lifting weights, working with resistance bands, or using body weight for resistance (such as push-ups, pull-ups, and sit-ups). Muscle-strengthening activities count if they involve a moderate to high level of effort and work the major muscle groups of the body: legs, hips, back, abdomen, chest, shoulders, and arms.

Levels of Intensity for Aerobic Activity

Children and adolescents can meet the Guidelines by doing a combination of moderate- and vigorous-intensity aerobic physical activities or by doing only vigorous-intensity aerobic physical activities.

Youth should not do only moderate-intensity activity. It's important to include vigorous-intensity activities because they cause more improvement in cardiorespiratory fitness.

The intensity of aerobic physical activity can be defined on either an absolute or a relative scale. Either scale can be used to monitor the intensity of aerobic physical activity:

- **Absolute intensity** is based on the rate of energy expenditure during the activity, without taking into account a person's cardiorespiratory fitness.

- **Relative intensity** uses a person's level of cardiorespiratory fitness to assess level of effort.

For More Information

See Appendix 1 for more information on using absolute or relative intensity.

Relative intensity describes a person's level of effort relative to his or her fitness. As a rule of thumb, on a scale of 0 to 10, where sitting is 0 and the highest level of effort possible is 10, moderate-intensity activity is a 5 or 6. Young people doing moderate-intensity activity will notice that their hearts are beating faster than normal and they are breathing harder than normal. Vigorous-intensity activity is at a level of 7 or 8. Youth doing vigorous-intensity activity will feel their heart beating much faster than normal and they will breathe much harder than normal.

When adults supervise children, they generally can't ascertain a child's heart or breathing rate. But they can observe whether a child is doing an activity which, based on absolute energy expenditure, is considered to be either moderate or vigorous. For example, a child walking briskly to school is doing moderate-intensity activity. A child running on the playground is doing vigorous-intensity activity. The table on page 18 includes examples of activities classified by absolute intensity. It shows that the same activity can be moderate or vigorous intensity, depending on factors such as speed (for example bicycling slowly or fast).

Physical Activity and Healthy Weight

Regular physical activity in children and adolescents promotes a healthy body weight and body composition.

Examples of Moderate- and Vigorous-Intensity Aerobic Physical Activities and Muscle- and Bone-Strengthening Activities for Children and Adolescents

Type of Physical Activity	Age Group	
	Children	Adolescents
Moderate–intensity aerobic	• Active recreation, such as hiking, skateboarding, rollerblading • Bicycle riding • Brisk walking	• Active recreation, such as canoeing, hiking, skateboarding, rollerblading • Brisk walking • Bicycle riding (stationary or road bike) • Housework and yard work, such as sweeping or pushing a lawn mower • Games that require catching and throwing, such as baseball and softball
Vigorous–intensity aerobic	• Active games involving running and chasing, such as tag • Bicycle riding • Jumping rope • Martial arts, such as karate • Running • Sports such as soccer, ice or field hockey, basketball, swimming, tennis • Cross-country skiing	• Active games involving running and chasing, such as flag football • Bicycle riding • Jumping rope • Martial arts, such as karate • Running • Sports such as soccer, ice or field hockey, basketball, swimming, tennis • Vigorous dancing • Cross-country skiing
Muscle-strengthening	• Games such as tug-of-war • Modified push-ups (with knees on the floor) • Resistance exercises using body weight or resistance bands • Rope or tree climbing • Sit-ups (curl-ups or crunches) • Swinging on playground equipment/bars	• Games such as tug-of-war • Push-ups and pull-ups • Resistance exercises with exercise bands, weight machines, hand-held weights • Climbing wall • Sit-ups (curl-ups or crunches)
Bone-strengthening	• Games such as hopscotch • Hopping, skipping, jumping • Jumping rope • Running • Sports such as gymnastics, basketball, volleyball, tennis	• Hopping, skipping, jumping • Jumping rope • Running • Sports such as gymnastics, basketball, volleyball, tennis

Note: Some activities, such as bicycling, can be moderate or vigorous intensity, depending upon level of effort

Exercise training in overweight or obese youth can improve body composition by reducing overall levels of fatness as well as abdominal fatness. Research studies report that fatness can be reduced by regular physical activity of moderate to vigorous intensity 3 to 5 times a week, for 30 to 60 minutes.

Meeting the Guidelines

American youth vary in their physical activity participation. Some don't participate at all, others participate in enough activity to meet the Guidelines, and some exceed the Guidelines.

Children and adolescents

can meet the Physical Activity Guidelines and become regularly physically active in many ways.

One practical strategy to promote activity in youth is to replace inactivity with activity whenever possible. For example, where appropriate and safe, young people should walk or bicycle to school instead of riding in a car. Rather than just watching sporting events on television, young people should participate in age-appropriate sports or games.

- **Children and adolescents who do not meet the Guidelines** should slowly increase their activity in small steps and in ways that they enjoy. A gradual increase in the number of days and the time spent being active will help reduce the risk of injury.

- **Children and adolescents who meet the Guidelines** should continue being active on a daily basis and, if appropriate, become even more active. Evidence suggests that even more than 60 minutes of activity every day may provide additional health benefits.

- **Children and adolescents who exceed the Guidelines** should maintain their activity level and vary the kinds of activities they do to reduce the risk of overtraining or injury.

Children and adolescents with disabilities are more likely to be inactive than those without disabilities. Youth with disabilities should work with their health-care provider to understand the types and amounts of physical activity appropriate for them. When possible, children and adolescents with disabilities should meet the Guidelines. When young people are not able to participate in appropriate physical activities to meet the Guidelines, they should be as active as possible and avoid being inactive.

Getting and Staying Active: Real-Life Examples

Children and adolescents can meet the Physical Activity Guidelines and become regularly physically active in many ways. Here are just two examples showing how a child and an adolescent can be physically active for at least 60 minutes each day over the course of a week.

These examples illustrate that even though the activity patterns are different, each young person is meeting the Guidelines by getting the equivalent of at least 60 minutes or more of aerobic activity each day that is at least moderate intensity. Both are also doing vigorous-intensity, muscle-strengthening, and bone-strengthening activities on at least 3 days a week.

Harold: A 7-Year-Old Child

Harold participates in many types of physical activities in many places. For example, during physical education class, he jumps rope and does gymnastics and sit-ups. During recess, he plays on the playground—often by doing activities that require running and climbing. He also likes to play soccer with his friends and family. When Harold gets home from school, he likes to engage in active play (playing tag) and ride his bicycle with his friends and family.

Harold gets 60 minutes of physical activity each day that is at least moderate intensity. He participates in the following activities each day:

Monday: Walks to and from school (20 minutes), plays actively with family (20 minutes), jumps rope (10 minutes), does gymnastics (10 minutes).

Tuesday: Walks to and from school (20 minutes), plays on playground (25 minutes), climbs on playground equipment (15 minutes).

Wednesday: Walks to and from school (20 minutes), plays actively with friends (25 minutes), jumps rope (10 minutes), runs (5 minutes), does sit-ups (2 minutes).

Thursday: Plays actively with family (30 minutes), plays soccer (30 minutes).

Friday: Walks to and from school (20 minutes), plays actively with friends (25 minutes), bicycles (15 minutes).

Saturday: Plays on playground (30 minutes), climbs on playground equipment (15 minutes), bicycles (15 minutes).

Sunday: Plays on playground (10 minutes), plays soccer (40 minutes), plays tag with family (10 minutes).

Harold meets the Guidelines by doing vigorous-intensity aerobic activities, bone-strengthening activities, and muscle-strengthening activities on at least 3 days of the week:

- **Vigorous-intensity** aerobic activities 6 times during the week: jumping rope (Monday and Wednesday), running (Wednesday), soccer (Thursday and Sunday), playing tag (Sunday);

- **Bone-strengthening** activities 6 times during the week: jumping rope (Monday and Wednesday), running (Wednesday), soccer (Thursday and Sunday), playing tag (Sunday); and

- **Muscle-strengthening** activities 4 times during the week: gymnastics (Monday), climbing on playground equipment (Tuesday and Saturday), sit-ups (Wednesday).

Maria: A 16-Year-Old Adolescent

Maria participates in many types of physical activities in many places. For example, during physical education class, she plays tennis and does sit-ups and push-ups. She also likes to play basketball at the YMCA, do yoga, and go dancing with friends. Maria likes to take her dog on walks and hikes.

Maria gets 60 or more minutes of daily physical activity that is at least moderate intensity. She participates in the following activities each day:

Monday: Walks dog (10 minutes), plays basketball at YMCA (50 minutes).

Tuesday: Walks dog (10 minutes), plays tennis (30 minutes), does sit-ups and push-ups (5 minutes), walks briskly with friends (15 minutes).

Wednesday: Walks dog (10 minutes), plays basketball at YMCA (50 minutes).

Thursday: Walks dog (10 minutes), plays tennis (30 minutes), does sit-ups and push-ups (5 minutes), plays with children at the park while babysitting (15 minutes).

Friday: Plays Frisbee® in park (45 minutes), mows lawn (30 minutes).

Saturday: Goes dancing with friends (60 minutes), does yoga (30 minutes).

Sunday: Hikes (60 minutes).

Maria meets the Guidelines by doing vigorous-intensity aerobic activities, bone-strengthening activities, and muscle-strengthening activities on at least 3 days of the week:

- **Vigorous-intensity** aerobic activities 4 times during the week: basketball (Monday and Wednesday), dancing (Saturday), hiking (Sunday);

- **Bone-strengthening** activities 4 times during the week: basketball (Monday and Wednesday), dancing (Saturday), hiking (Sunday); and

- **Muscle-strengthening** activities 3 times during the week: sit-ups and push-ups (Tuesday and Thursday), yoga (Saturday).

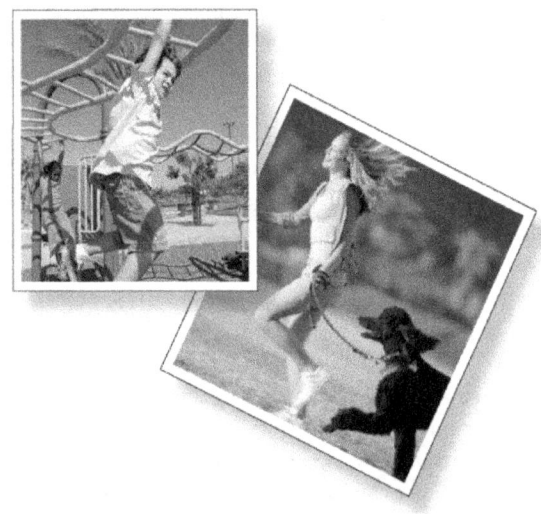

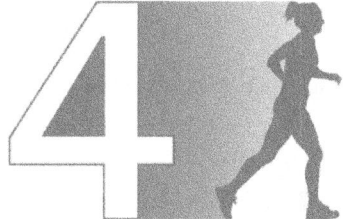

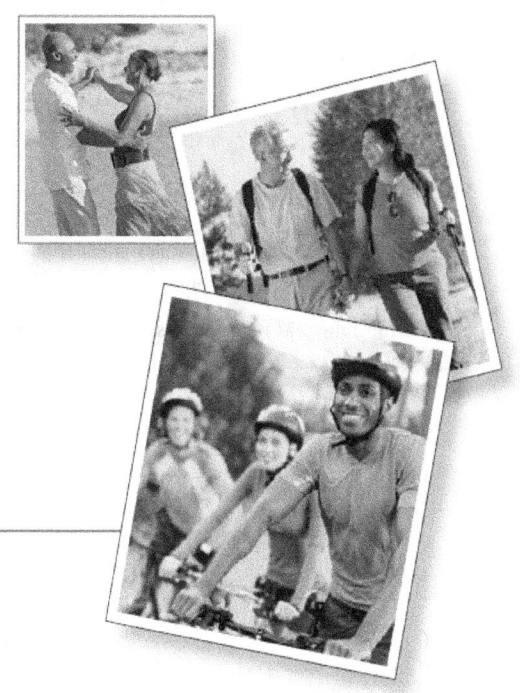

Active Adults

A dults who are physically active are healthier and less likely to develop many chronic diseases than adults who are inactive. They also have better fitness, including a healthier body size and composition. These benefits are gained by men and women and people of all races and ethnicities who have been studied.

Adults gain most of these health benefits when they do the equivalent of at least 150 minutes of moderate-intensity aerobic physical activity (2 hours and 30 minutes) each week. Adults gain additional and more extensive health and fitness benefits with even more physical activity. Muscle-strengthening activities also provide health benefits and are an important part of an adult's overall physical activity plan.

This chapter provides guidance for most men and women aged 18 to 64 years, and focuses on physical activity beyond baseline activity (the usual light or sedentary activities of daily living). Physical activity guidelines for women during pregnancy and the postpartum period and for adults with disabilities and select chronic conditions are discussed in Chapter 7—Additional Considerations for Some Adults.

Explaining the Guidelines

The Guidelines for adults focus on two types of activity: aerobic and muscle-strengthening. Each type provides important health benefits, as explained in Chapter 2—Physical Activity Has Many Health Benefits.

Aerobic Activity

Aerobic activities, also called endurance activities, are physical activities in which people move their large muscles in a rhythmic manner for a sustained period. Running, brisk walking, bicycling, playing basketball, dancing, and swimming are all examples of aerobic activities. Aerobic activity makes a person's heart beat more rapidly to meet the demands of the body's movement. Over time, regular aerobic activity makes the heart and cardiovascular system stronger and fitter.

The purpose of the aerobic activity does not affect whether it counts toward meeting the Guidelines. For example, physically active occupations can count toward meeting the Guidelines, as can active transportation choices (walking or bicycling). All types of aerobic activities can count as long as they are of

Key Guidelines for Adults

- All adults should avoid inactivity. Some physical activity is better than none, and adults who participate in any amount of physical activity gain some health benefits.

- For substantial health benefits, adults should do at least 150 minutes (2 hours and 30 minutes) a week of moderate-intensity, or 75 minutes (1 hour and 15 minutes) a week of vigorous-intensity aerobic physical activity, or an equivalent combination of moderate- and vigorous-intensity aerobic activity. Aerobic activity should be performed in episodes of at least 10 minutes, and preferably, it should be spread throughout the week.

- For additional and more extensive health benefits, adults should increase their aerobic physical activity to 300 minutes (5 hours) a week of moderate-intensity, or 150 minutes a week of vigorous-intensity aerobic physical activity, or an equivalent combination of moderate- and vigorous-intensity activity. Additional health benefits are gained by engaging in physical activity beyond this amount.

- Adults should also do muscle-strengthening activities that are moderate or high intensity and involve all major muscle groups on 2 or more days a week, as these activities provide additional health benefits.

sufficient intensity and duration. Time spent in muscle-strengthening activities does not count toward the aerobic activity guidelines.

When putting the Guidelines into action, it's important to consider the total amount of activity, as well as how often to be active, for how long, and at what intensity.

How Much Total Activity a Week?

When adults do the equivalent of 150 minutes of moderate-intensity aerobic activity each week, the benefits are *substantial*. These benefits include lower risk of premature death, coronary heart disease, stroke, hypertension, type 2 diabetes, and depression.

Not all health benefits of physical activity occur at 150 minutes a week. As a person moves from 150 minutes a week toward 300 minutes (5 hours) a week, he or she gains *additional* health benefits. Additional benefits include lower risk of colon and breast cancer and prevention of unhealthy weight gain.

Also, as a person moves from 150 minutes a week toward 300 minutes a week, the benefits that occur at 150 minutes a week become *more extensive*. For example, a person who does 300 minutes a week has an even lower risk of heart disease or diabetes than a person who does 150 minutes a week.

The benefits continue to increase when a person does more than the equivalent of 300 minutes a week of moderate-intensity aerobic activity. For example, a person who does 420 minutes (7 hours) a week has an even lower risk of premature death than a person who does 150 to 300 minutes a week. Current science does not allow identifying an upper limit of total activity above which there are no additional health benefits.

How Many Days a Week and for How Long?

Aerobic physical activity should preferably be spread throughout the week. Research studies consistently show that activity performed on at least 3 days a week produces health benefits. Spreading physical activity across at least 3 days a week may help to reduce the risk of injury and avoid excessive fatigue.

Both moderate- and vigorous-intensity aerobic activity should be performed in episodes of at least 10 minutes. Episodes of this duration are known to improve cardiovascular fitness and some risk factors for heart disease and type 2 diabetes.

How Intense?

The Guidelines for adults focus on two levels of intensity: moderate-intensity activity and vigorous-intensity activity. To meet the Guidelines, adults can do either moderate-intensity or vigorous-intensity aerobic activities, or a combination of both. It takes less time to get the same benefit from vigorous-intensity activities as from moderate-intensity activities. A general rule of thumb is that 2 minutes of moderate-intensity activity counts the same as 1 minute of vigorous-intensity activity. For example, 30 minutes of moderate-intensity activity a week is roughly the same as 15 minutes of vigorous-intensity activity.

There are two ways to track the intensity of aerobic activity: absolute intensity and relative intensity.

- **Absolute intensity** is the amount of energy expended per minute of activity. The energy expenditure of light-intensity activity, for example, is 1.1 to 2.9 times the amount of energy expended when a person is at rest. Moderate-intensity activities expend 3.0 to 5.9 times the amount of energy expended at rest. The energy expenditure of vigorous-intensity activities is 6.0 or more times the energy expended at rest.

- **Relative intensity** is the level of effort required to do an activity. Less fit people generally require a higher level of effort than fitter people to do the same activity. Relative intensity can be estimated using a scale of 0 to 10, where sitting is 0 and the highest level of effort possible is 10. Moderate-intensity activity is a 5 or 6. Vigorous-intensity activity is a 7 or 8.

The Guidelines for adults refer to absolute intensity because most studies demonstrating lower risks of clinical events (for example, premature death, cardiovascular disease, type 2 diabetes, cancer) have focused on measuring absolute intensity. That is, the Guidelines are based on the absolute amount of energy expended in physical activity that is associated with health benefits. The table lists some examples of activities classified as moderate-intensity or vigorous-intensity based on absolute intensity. Either absolute or relative intensity can be used to monitor progress in meeting the Guidelines.

When using relative intensity, people pay attention to how physical activity affects their heart rate

For More Information

See Appendix 1 for more information on using absolute or relative intensity.

Examples of Different Aerobic Physical Activities and Intensities

Moderate Intensity
• Walking briskly (3 miles per hour or faster, but not race-walking)
• Water aerobics
• Bicycling slower than 10 miles per hour
• Tennis (doubles)
• Ballroom dancing
• General gardening

Vigorous Intensity
• Racewalking, jogging, or running
• Swimming laps
• Tennis (singles)
• Aerobic dancing
• Bicycling 10 miles per hour or faster
• Jumping rope
• Heavy gardening (continuous digging or hoeing, with heart rate increases)
• Hiking uphill or with a heavy backpack

Note: This table provides several examples of activities classified as moderate-intensity or vigorous-intensity, based on absolute intensity. This list is not all-inclusive. Instead, the examples are meant to help people make choices.

and breathing. As a rule of thumb, a person doing moderate-intensity aerobic activity can talk, but not sing, during the activity. A person doing vigorous-intensity activity cannot say more than a few words without pausing for a breath.

Muscle-Strengthening Activity

Muscle-strengthening activities provide additional benefits not found with aerobic activity. The benefits of muscle-strengthening activity include increased bone strength and muscular fitness. Muscle-strengthening activities can also help maintain muscle mass during a program of weight loss.

Muscle-strengthening activities make muscles do more work than they are accustomed to doing. That is, they overload the muscles. Resistance training, including weight training, is a familiar example of muscle-strengthening activity. Other examples include working with resistance bands, doing calisthenics that use body weight for resistance (such as push-ups, pull-ups, and sit-ups), carrying heavy loads, and heavy gardening (such as digging or hoeing).

Muscle-strengthening activities count if they involve a moderate to high level of intensity or effort and work the major muscle groups of the body: the legs, hips, back, chest, abdomen, shoulders, and arms. Muscle-strengthening activities for all the major muscle groups should be done at least 2 days a week.

No specific amount of time is recommended for muscle strengthening, but muscle-strengthening exercises should be performed to the point at which it would be difficult to do another repetition without help. When resistance training is used to enhance muscle strength, one set of 8 to 12 repetitions of each exercise is effective, although two or three sets may be more effective. Development of muscle strength and endurance is progressive over time. Increases in the amount of weight or the days a week of exercising will result in stronger muscles.

Meeting the Guidelines

Adults have many options for becoming physically active, increasing their physical activity, and staying active throughout their lives. In deciding how to meet the Guidelines, adults should think about how much physical activity they're already doing and how physically fit they are. Personal health and fitness goals are also important to consider. Examples provided later in the chapter illustrate how to include these goals in decisions to be active.

In general, healthy men and women who plan prudent increases in their weekly amounts of physical activity do not need to consult a health-care provider before becoming active.

Inactive Adults

Inactive adults or those who don't yet do 150 minutes of physical activity a week should work gradually toward this goal. The initial amount of activity should be at a light or moderate intensity, for short periods of time, with the sessions spread throughout the week. The good news is that "some is better than none."

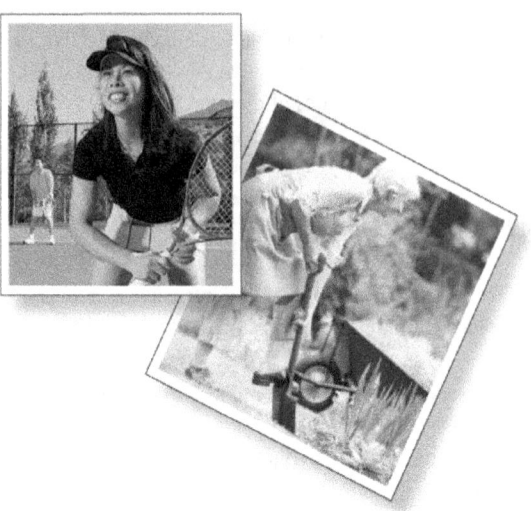

People gain some health benefits even when they do as little as 60 minutes a week of moderate-intensity aerobic physical activity.

To reduce risk of injury, it is important to increase the amount of physical activity gradually over a period of weeks to months.

For More Information

See Chapter 6—Safe and Active, for more information on how to increase physical activity gradually.

For example, an inactive person could start with a walking program consisting of 5 minutes of slow walking several times each day, 5 to 6 days a week. The length of time could then gradually be increased to 10 minutes per session, 3 times a day, and the walking speed could be increased slowly.

Muscle-strengthening activities should also be gradually increased over time. Initially, these activities can be done just 1 day a week starting at a light or moderate level of effort. Over time, the number of days a week can be increased to 2, and then possibly to more than 2. Each week, the level of effort (intensity) can be increased slightly until it becomes moderate to high.

Active Adults

Adults who are already active and meet the minimum Guidelines (the equivalent of 150 minutes of moderate-intensity aerobic activity every week) can gain additional and more extensive health and fitness benefits by increasing physical activity above this amount. Most American adults should increase their aerobic activity to exceed the minimum level and move toward 300 minutes a week. Adults should also do muscle-strengthening activities on at least 2 days each week.

One time-efficient way to achieve greater fitness and health goals is to substitute vigorous-intensity aerobic activity for some moderate-intensity activity. Using the 2-to-1 rule of thumb, doing 150 minutes of vigorous-intensity aerobic activity a week provides about the same benefits as 300 minutes of moderate-intensity activity.

Adults are encouraged to do a variety of activities, as variety probably reduces risk of injury caused by doing too much of one kind of activity (this is called an overuse injury).

Highly Active Adults

Adults who are highly active should maintain their activity level. These adults are also encouraged to do a variety of activities.

Special Considerations

Flexibility Activities

Flexibility is an important part of physical fitness. Some types of physical activity, such as dancing, require more flexibility than others. Stretching exercises are effective in increasing flexibility, and thereby can allow people to more easily do activities that require greater flexibility. For this reason, flexibility activities are an appropriate part of a physical activity program, even though they have no known health benefits and it is unclear whether they reduce risk of injury. Time spent doing flexibility activities by themselves does not count toward meeting the aerobic or muscle-strengthening Guidelines.

Warm-up and Cool-down

Warm-up and cool-down activities are an acceptable part of a person's physical activity plan. Commonly, the warm-up and cool-down involve doing an activity at a slower speed or lower intensity. A warm-up before moderate- or vigorous-intensity aerobic activity allows a gradual increase in heart rate and breathing at the start of the episode of activity. A cool-down after activity allows a gradual decrease at the end of the episode. Time spent doing warm-up and cool-down may count toward meeting the aerobic activity Guidelines if the activity is at least moderate intensity (for example, walking briskly as a warm-up before jogging). A warm-up for muscle-strengthening activity commonly involves doing exercises with lighter weight.

Physical Activity in a Weight-Control Plan

Along with appropriate dietary intake, physical activity is an important part of maintaining healthy weight, losing weight, and keeping extra weight off once it has been lost. Physical activity also helps reduce abdominal fat and preserve muscle during weight loss. Adults should aim for a healthy, stable body weight. The amount of physical activity necessary to achieve this weight varies greatly from person to person.

> **For More Information**
>
> See the *Dietary Guidelines for Americans* for additional information on weight management and how to determine a healthy weight.

The first step in achieving or maintaining a healthy weight is to meet the minimum level of physical activity in the Guidelines. For some people this will result in a stable and healthy body weight, but for many it may not.

The health benefits

of physical activity are generally independent of body weight. The good news for people needing to lose weight is that regular physical activity provides major health benefits, no matter how their weight changes over time.

Adults should

strongly consider walking as one good way to get aerobic physical activity. Many studies show that walking has health benefits and a low risk of injury. It can be done year-round and in many settings.

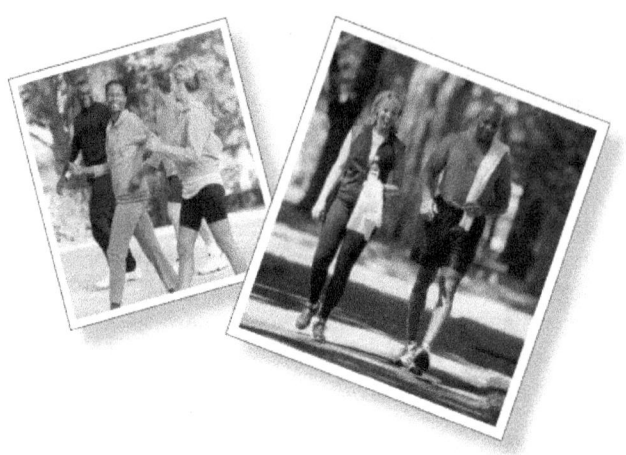

People who are at a healthy body weight but slowly gaining weight can either gradually increase the level of physical activity (toward the equivalent of 300 minutes a week of moderate-intensity aerobic activity), or reduce caloric intake, or both, until their weight is stable. By regularly checking body weight, people can find the amount of physical activity that works for them.

Many adults will need to do more than the 150 minutes a week of moderate-intensity aerobic physical activity as part of a program to lose weight or keep it off. These adults should do more physical activity and/or further reduce their caloric intake. Some people will need to do the equivalent of 300 or more minutes of moderate-intensity physical activity a week to meet their weight-control goals. Combined with restricting caloric intake, these adults should gradually increase minutes or the intensity of aerobic physical activity per week, to the point at which the physical activity is effective in achieving a healthy weight.

It is important to remember that all activities—both baseline and physical activity—"count" for energy balance. Active choices, such as taking the stairs rather than the elevator or adding short episodes of walking to the day, are examples of activities that can be helpful in weight control.

For weight control, vigorous-intensity activity is far more time-efficient than moderate-intensity activity. For example, an adult who weighs 165 pounds (75 kg) will burn 560 calories from 150 minutes of brisk walking at 4 miles an hour (these calories are in addition to the calories normally burned by a body at rest). That person can burn the same number of additional calories in 50 minutes by running 5 miles at a 10 minutes-per-mile pace.

Getting and Staying Active: Real-Life Examples

Adults can meet the *Physical Activity Guidelines* in all sorts of ways and with many types of physical activity. The choices of types and amounts of physical activity depend on personal health and fitness goals. Here are three examples.

Jean: An Inactive Middle-Aged Woman

Her goals: Jean sets a goal of doing 1 hour a day of moderate-intensity aerobic activity on 5 days a week (a total of 300 minutes a week). Weighing 220 pounds, Jean is obese and wants to lose about 1 pound of weight each week.

Starting out: Jean cuts back on her caloric intake and starts walking 5 minutes in the morning and 5 minutes in the evening most days of the week. She walks at a 2.5 mile-an-hour pace. Although physical activity tables show this to be light-intensity activity, for her level of fitness and fatness, it is appropriate moderate-intensity activity.

Making good progress: Two months later, Jean is comfortably walking 30 to 40 minutes at moderate intensity to and from her bus stop every day. She then adds variety to her activity by alternating among walking, riding a stationary cycle, and low-impact aerobics. She also begins muscle-strengthening activities, using elastic bands twice each week.

Adults can meet

the *Physical Activity Guidelines* in all sorts of ways and with many types of physical activity.

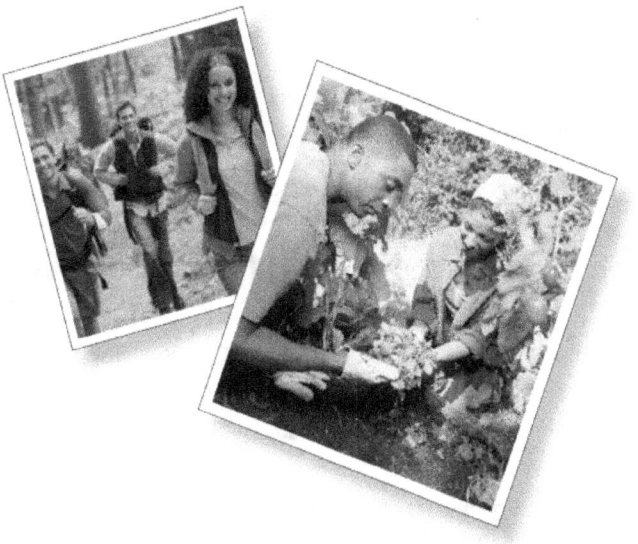

Reaching her goal: Eventually, Jean works up to 300 minutes a week of moderate-intensity aerobic activity, including her brisk walks to and from the bus stop. She has lost 40 pounds of weight in 1 year, with most of the weight loss occurring the previous 6 months when she mastered her diet and was able to do greater amounts of physical activity.

Douglas: An Active Middle-Aged Man

His goal and current activity pattern: Douglas was a soccer player in his youth. His goal is to get back into shape by becoming a regular recreational runner. In addition to his job operating heavy equipment, he walks 30 to 40 minutes a day on 5 days each week. He also lifts weights 2 days a week.

Starting out: Douglas starts a walk/jog program with a co-worker and plans to gradually replace walking with jogging and then running. The first week he goes out on 5 days, walking for 25 minutes and jogging for 5 minutes.

Making good progress: Each week, Douglas gradually increases the time spent jogging (vigorous-intensity activity) and reduces the time spent walking (moderate-intensity activity). He also continues his weight-lifting program.

Reaching his goal: Eventually, Douglas is running 30 to 45 minutes 4 days a week and lifting weights

2 days a week. He goes for a 1-hour bicycle ride on most weekends.

Anita: A Very Active College-Aged Adult

Her goals and current activity pattern: Anita plays league basketball (vigorous-intensity activity) 4 days each week for 90 minutes each day. She wants to reduce her risk of injury from doing too much of one kind of activity (this is called an overuse injury).

Starting out: Anita starts out by cutting back her basketball playing to 3 days each week. She begins to bicycle to and from campus (30 minutes each way) instead of driving her car. She also joins a yoga class that meets twice each week.

Reaching her goal: Eventually, Anita is bicycling 3 days each week to and from campus in addition to playing basketball. Her yoga class helps her to build and maintain strength and flexibility.

Achieving Target Levels of Physical Activity: The Possibilities Are Endless

These examples show how it's possible to meet the Guidelines by doing moderate-intensity or vigorous-intensity activity or a combination of both. Physical activity at this level provides substantial health benefits.

Ways to get the equivalent of 150 minutes (2 hours and 30 minutes) of moderate-intensity aerobic physical activity a week plus muscle-strengthening activities:

- Thirty minutes of brisk walking (moderate intensity) on 5 days, exercising with resistance bands (muscle strengthening) on 2 days;

- Twenty-five minutes of running (vigorous intensity) on 3 days, lifting weights on 2 days (muscle strengthening);

- Thirty minutes of brisk walking on 2 days, 60 minutes (1 hour) of social dancing (moderate intensity) on 1 evening, 30 minutes of mowing the lawn (moderate intensity) on 1 afternoon, heavy gardening (muscle strengthening) on 2 days;

- Thirty minutes of an aerobic dance class on 1 morning (vigorous intensity), 30 minutes of running on 1 day (vigorous intensity), 30 minutes of brisk walking on 1 day (moderate intensity), calisthenics (such as sit-ups, push-ups) on 3 days (muscle strengthening);

- Thirty minutes of biking to and from work on 3 days (moderate intensity), playing softball for 60 minutes on 1 day (moderate intensity), using weight machines on 2 days (muscle-strengthening on 2 days); and

- Forty-five minutes of doubles tennis on 2 days (moderate intensity), lifting weights after work on 1 day (muscle strengthening), hiking vigorously for 30 minutes and rock climbing (muscle strengthening) on 1 day.

Ways to be even more active

For adults who are already doing at least 150 minutes of moderate-intensity physical activity, here are a few ways to do even more. Physical activity at this level has even greater health benefits.

- Forty-five minutes of brisk walking every day, exercising with resistance bands on 2 or 3 days;

- Forty-five minutes of running on 3 or 4 days, circuit weight training in a gym on 2 or 3 days;

- Thirty minutes of running on 2 days, 45 minutes of brisk walking on 1 day, 45 minutes of an aerobics and weights class on 1 day, 90 minutes (1 hour and 30 minutes) of social dancing on 1 evening, 30 minutes of mowing the lawn, plus some heavy garden work on 1 day;

- Ninety minutes of playing soccer on 1 day, brisk walking for 15 minutes on 3 days, lifting weights on 2 days; and

- Forty-five minutes of stationary bicycling on 2 days, 60 minutes of basketball on 2 days, calisthenics on 3 days.

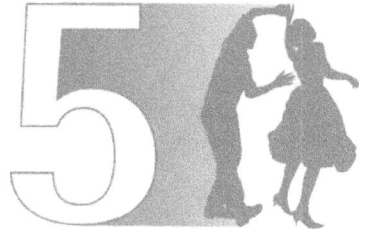

Active Older Adults

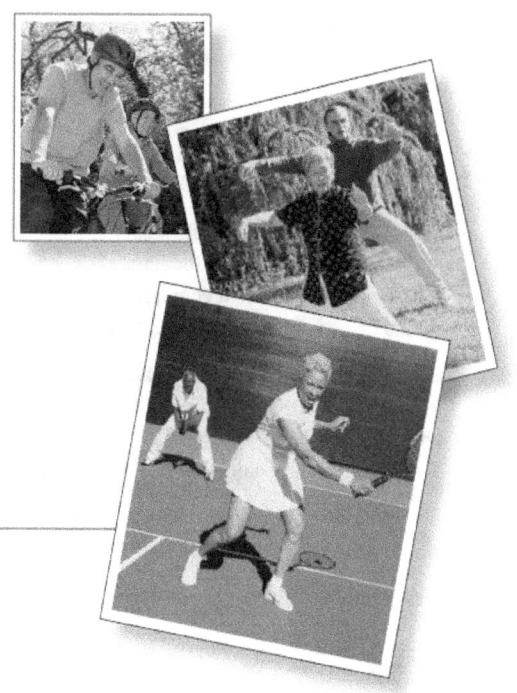

Regular physical activity is essential for healthy aging. Adults aged 65 years and older gain substantial health benefits from regular physical activity, and these benefits continue to occur throughout their lives. Promoting physical activity for older adults is especially important because this population is the least physically active of any age group.

Older adults are a varied group. Most, but not all, have one or more chronic conditions, and these conditions vary in type and severity. All have experienced a loss of physical fitness with age, some more than others. This diversity means that some older adults can run several miles, while others struggle to walk several blocks.

This chapter provides guidance about physical activity for adults aged 65 years and older. The chapter focuses on physical activity beyond baseline activity. The Guidelines seek to help older adults select types and amounts of physical activity appropriate for their abilities. The Guidelines for older adults are also appropriate for adults younger than age 65 who have chronic conditions and those with a low level of fitness.

For adults aged 65 and older who are fit and have no limiting chronic conditions, the guidance in this chapter is essentially the same as that provided in Chapter 4–Active Adults.

Explaining the Guidelines

Like the Guidelines for other adults, those for older adults mainly focus on two types of activity: aerobic and muscle-strengthening. In addition, these Guidelines discuss the addition of balance training for older adults at risk of falls. Each type provides important health benefits, as explained in Chapter 2–Physical Activity Has Many Health Benefits.

Aerobic Activity

People doing aerobic activities move large muscles in a rhythmic manner for a sustained period. Brisk walking, jogging, biking, dancing, and swimming are all examples of aerobic activities. This type of activity is also called endurance activity.

Aerobic activity makes a person's heart beat more rapidly to meet the demands of the body's movement.

Key Guidelines for Older Adults

The following Guidelines are the same for adults and older adults:

- All older adults should avoid inactivity. Some physical activity is better than none, and older adults who participate in any amount of physical activity gain some health benefits.

- For substantial health benefits, older adults should do at least 150 minutes (2 hours and 30 minutes) a week of moderate-intensity, or 75 minutes (1 hour and 15 minutes) a week of vigorous-intensity aerobic physical activity, or an equivalent combination of moderate- and vigorous-intensity aerobic activity. Aerobic activity should be performed in episodes of at least 10 minutes, and preferably, it should be spread throughout the week.

- For additional and more extensive health benefits, older adults should increase their aerobic physical activity to 300 minutes (5 hours) a week of moderate-intensity, or 150 minutes a week of vigorous-intensity aerobic physical activity, or an equivalent combination of moderate- and vigorous-intensity activity. Additional health benefits are gained by engaging in physical activity beyond this amount.

- Older adults should also do muscle-strengthening activities that are moderate or high intensity and involve all major muscle groups on 2 or more days a week, as these activities provide additional health benefits.

The following Guidelines are just for older adults:

- When older adults cannot do 150 minutes of moderate-intensity aerobic activity a week because of chronic conditions, they should be as physically active as their abilities and conditions allow.

- Older adults should do exercises that maintain or improve balance if they are at risk of falling.

- Older adults should determine their level of effort for physical activity relative to their level of fitness.

- Older adults with chronic conditions should understand whether and how their conditions affect their ability to do regular physical activity safely.

Over time, regular aerobic activity makes the heart and cardiovascular system stronger and fitter.

When putting the Guidelines into action, it's important to consider the total amount of activity, as well as how often to be active, for how long, and at what intensity.

How much total activity a week?

Older adults should aim to do at least 150 minutes (2 hours and 30 minutes) of moderate-intensity physical activity a week, or an equivalent amount (75 minutes or 1 hour and 15 minutes) of vigorous-intensity activity. Older adults can also do an equivalent amount of activity by combining moderate- and vigorous-intensity activity. As is true for younger people, greater amounts of physical activity provide additional and more extensive health benefits to people aged 65 years and older.

No matter what its purpose—walking the dog, taking a dance or exercise class, or bicycling to the store—aerobic activity of all types counts toward the Guidelines.

How many days a week and for how long?

Aerobic physical activity should be spread throughout the week. Research studies consistently show that activity performed on at least 3 days a week produces health benefits. Spreading physical activity across at least 3 days a week may help to reduce the risk of injury and avoid excessive fatigue.

Episodes of aerobic activity count toward meeting the Guidelines if they last at least 10 minutes and are performed at moderate or vigorous intensity. These episodes can be divided throughout the day or week. For example, a person who takes a brisk 15-minute

Examples of Aerobic and Muscle-Strengthening Physical Activities for Older Adults

The intensity of these activities can be either relatively moderate or relatively vigorous, depending on an older adult's level of fitness.

Aerobic	Muscle-Strengthening
• Walking	• Exercises using exercise bands, weight machines, hand-held weights
• Dancing	
• Swimming	
• Water aerobics	• Calisthenic exercises (body weight provides resistance to movement)
• Jogging	
• Aerobic exercise classes	
• Bicycle riding (stationary or on a path)	• Digging, lifting, and carrying as part of gardening
• Some activities of gardening, such as raking and pushing a lawn mower	• Carrying groceries
	• Some yoga exercises
• Tennis	• Some tai chi exercises
• Golf (without a cart)	

walk twice a day on every day of the week would easily meet the minimum Guideline for aerobic activity.

How intense?

Older adults can meet the Guidelines by doing relatively moderate-intensity activity, relatively vigorous-intensity activity, or a combination of both. Time spent in light activity (such as light housework) and sedentary activities (such as watching TV) do not count.

The relative intensity of aerobic activity is related to a person's level of cardiorespiratory fitness.

• **Moderate-intensity activity** requires a medium level of effort. On a scale of 0 to 10, where sitting is 0 and the greatest effort possible is 10, moderate-intensity activity is a 5 or 6 and produces noticeable increases in breathing rate and heart rate.

• **Vigorous-intensity activity** is a 7 or 8 on this scale and produces large increases in a person's breathing and heart rate.

A general rule of thumb is that 2 minutes of moderate-intensity activity count the same as 1 minute of vigorous-intensity activity. For example, 30 minutes of moderate-intensity activity a week is roughly same as 15 minutes of vigorous-intensity activity.

Muscle-Strengthening Activities

At least 2 days a week, older adults should do muscle-strengthening activities that involve all the major muscle groups. These are the muscles of the legs, hips, chest, back, abdomen, shoulders, and arms.

Muscle-strengthening activities make muscles do more work than they are accustomed to during activities of daily life. Examples of muscle-strengthening activities include lifting weights, working with resistance bands, doing calisthenics using body weight for resistance (such as push-ups, pull-ups, and sit-ups), climbing stairs, carrying heavy loads, and heavy gardening.

Muscle-strengthening activities count if they involve a moderate to high level of intensity, or effort, and work the major muscle groups of the body. Whatever the reason for doing it, any muscle-strengthening activity counts toward meeting the Guidelines. For example, muscle-strengthening activity done as part of a therapy or rehabilitation program can count.

No specific amount of time is recommended for muscle strengthening, but muscle-strengthening exercises should be performed to the point at which it would be difficult to do another repetition without help. When resistance training is used to enhance muscle strength, one set of 8 to 12 repetitions of each exercise is effective, although two or three sets may be more effective. Development of muscle strength and endurance is progressive over time. This means that gradual increases in the amount of weight or the days per week of exercise will result in stronger muscles.

Balance Activities for Older Adults at Risk of Falls

Older adults are at increased risk of falls if they have had falls in the recent past or have trouble walking. In older adults at increased risk of falls, strong evidence shows that regular physical activity is safe and reduces the risk of falls. Reduction in falls is seen for participants in programs that include balance and moderate-intensity muscle-strengthening activities for 90 minutes (1 hour and 30 minutes) a week plus moderate-intensity walking for about 1 hour a week. Preferably, older adults at risk of falls should do balance training 3 or more days a week and do standardized exercises from a program demonstrated to reduce falls. Examples of these exercises include backward walking, sideways walking, heel walking, toe walking, and standing from a sitting position. The exercises can increase in difficulty by progressing from holding onto a stable support (like furniture) while doing the exercises to doing them without support. It's not known whether different combinations of type, amount, or frequency of activity can reduce falls to a greater degree. Tai chi exercises also may help prevent falls.

Meeting the Guidelines

Older adults have many ways to live an active lifestyle that meets the Guidelines. Many factors influence decisions to be active, such as personal goals, current physical activity habits, and health and safety considerations.

Healthy older adults generally do not need to consult a health-care provider before becoming physically active. However, health-care providers can help people attain and maintain regular physical activity by providing advice on appropriate types of activities and ways to progress at a safe and steady pace.

For More Information

See Chapter 6—Safe and Active, for details on consulting a health-care provider.

Adults with chronic conditions should talk with their health-care provider to determine whether their conditions limit their ability to do regular physical activity in any way. Such a conversation should also help people learn about appropriate types and amounts of physical activity.

Inactive Older Adults

Older adults should increase their amount of physical activity gradually. It can take months for those with a low level of fitness to gradually meet their activity goals. To reduce injury risk, inactive or insufficiently active adults should avoid vigorous aerobic activity at first. Rather, they should gradually increase the number of days a week and duration of moderate-intensity aerobic activity. Adults with a very low level of fitness can start out with episodes of activity less than 10 minutes and slowly increase the minutes of light-intensity aerobic activity, such as light-intensity walking.

Older adults who are inactive or who don't yet meet the Guidelines should aim for at least 150 minutes a week of relatively moderate-intensity physical activity. Getting at least 30 minutes of relatively moderate-intensity physical activity on 5 or more days each week is a reasonable way to meet these Guidelines. Doing muscle-strengthening activity on 2 or 3 non-consecutive days each week is also an acceptable and appropriate goal for many older adults.

Active Older Adults

Older adults who are already active and meet the Guidelines can gain additional and more extensive health benefits by moving beyond the 150-minute-a-week minimum to 300 or more minutes a week of relatively moderate-intensity aerobic activity. Muscle-strengthening activities should also be done at least 2 days a week.

Older Adults With Chronic Conditions

Older adults who have chronic conditions that prevent them from doing the equivalent of 150 minutes of moderate-intensity aerobic activity a week should set physical activity goals that meet their abilities. They should talk with their health-care provider about setting physical activity goals. They should avoid an inactive lifestyle. Even 60 minutes (1 hour) a week of moderate-intensity aerobic activity provides some health benefits.

For More Information

See Chapter 7—Additional Considerations for Some Adults, for more information on chronic conditions.

Special Considerations
Doing a Variety of Activities, Including Walking

In working toward meeting the Guidelines, older adults are encouraged to do a variety of activities. This

Older adults

have many ways to live an active
lifestyle that meets the Guidelines.

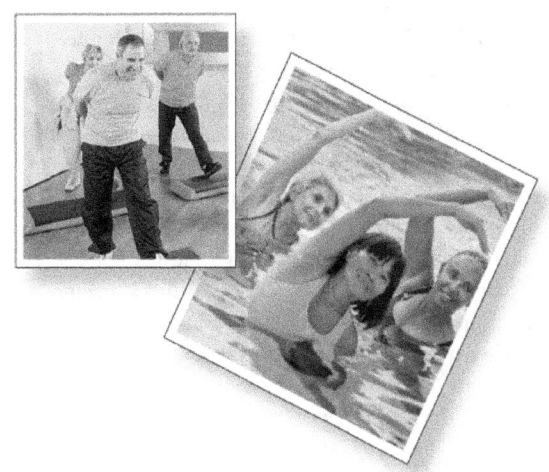

approach can make activity more enjoyable and may
reduce the risk of overuse injury.

Older adults also should strongly consider walking as
one good way to get aerobic activity. Many studies show
that walking has health benefits, and it has a low risk of
injury. It can be done year-round and in many settings.

Physical Activity for Older Adults Who Have Functional Limitations

When a person has lost some ability to do a task of
everyday life, such as climbing stairs, the person has
a functional limitation. In older adults with existing
functional limitations, scientific evidence indicates
that regular physical activity is safe and helps improve
functional ability.

Resuming Activity After an Illness or Injury

Older adults may have to take a break from regular
physical activity because of illness or injury, such as
the flu or a muscle strain. If these interruptions occur,
older adults should resume activity at a lower level and
gradually work back up to their former level of activity.

Flexibility, Warm-up, and Cool-down

Older adults should maintain the flexibility necessary
for regular physical activity and activities of daily
life. When done properly, stretching activities increase
flexibility. Although these activities alone have no
known health benefits and have not been demonstrated
to reduce risk of activity-related injuries, they are an
appropriate component of a physical activity program.
However, time spent doing flexibility activities by
themselves does not count toward meeting aerobic or
muscle-strengthening Guidelines.

Research studies of effective exercise programs
typically include warm-up and cool-down activities.
Warm-up and cool-down activities before and after

physical activity can also be included as part of a
personal program. A warm-up before moderate- or
vigorous-intensity aerobic activity allows a gradual
increase in heart rate and breathing at the start of
the episode of activity. A cool-down after activity
allows a gradual decrease at the end of the episode.
Time spent doing warm-up and cool-down may count
toward meeting the aerobic activity Guidelines if the
activity is at least moderate intensity (for example,
walking briskly to warm-up for a jog). A warm-up
for muscle-strengthening activity commonly involves
doing exercises with less weight than during the
strengthening activity.

Physical Activity in a Weight-Control Plan

The amount of physical activity necessary to
successfully maintain a healthy body weight depends
on caloric intake and varies considerably among
older adults. To achieve and maintain a healthy body
weight, older adults should first do the equivalent of
150 minutes of moderate-intensity aerobic activity each
week. If necessary, older adults should increase their
weekly minutes of aerobic physical activity gradually
over time and decrease caloric intake to a point where
they can achieve energy balance and a healthy weight.

Some older adults will need a higher level of physical
activity than others to maintain a healthy body
weight. Some may need more than the equivalent of
300 minutes (5 hours) a week of moderate-intensity
activity. It is possible to achieve this level of activity by
gradually increasing activity over time.

Older adults who are capable of relatively vigorous-intensity activity and need a high level of physical activity to maintain a healthy weight should consider some relatively vigorous-intensity activity as a means of weight control. This approach is more time-efficient than doing only moderate-intensity activity. However, high levels of activity are not feasible for many older adults. These adults should achieve a level of physical activity that is sustainable and safe. If further weight loss is needed, these older adults should achieve energy balance by regulating caloric intake.

It is important to remember that all activities "count" for energy balance. Active choices, such as taking the stairs rather than the elevator or adding short episodes of walking to the day, are examples of activities that can be helpful in weight control.

Getting and Staying Active: Real-Life Examples

The following examples show how different people with different living circumstances and levels of fitness can meet the Guidelines for older adults.

Mary: A 75-Year-Old Woman Living Independently in Her Own Home

Mary gets the equivalent of 180 minutes (3 hours) of moderate-intensity aerobic activity each week, plus muscle-strengthening activity 3 days a week.

- She participates regularly in an exercise class at her local senior center. The class meets Mondays, Wednesdays, and Fridays. It includes 30 minutes of aerobic dance, which she can do at moderate intensity, as well as 20 minutes of strength training, a 5-minute warm-up, a 5-minute cool-down, and some stretching exercises.

- On most Sundays, she visits her favorite park and walks a loop trail with several friends, which takes them about 45 minutes. The trail is hilly, so about 30 minutes of the walk is moderate-intensity walking for her, and about 15 minutes is vigorous-intensity (the 15 minutes of vigorous intensity counts as 30 minutes of moderate-intensity walking).

- She adds at least an additional 30 minutes of walking each week in different ways. For example, she walks

her grandson to school, she walks to her friends' homes, or she walks at the mall during shopping trips.

Manuel: An 85-Year-Old Man Living in an Assisted-Living Facility

Manuel, who has problems with falls, gets about 70 minutes (1 hour and 10 minutes) of aerobic activity each week and has an individualized strength-training program. He cannot do 150 minutes of moderate-intensity physical activity because of his chronic conditions, but he is being as physically active as his condition allows.

- To reduce the risk of falls, a physical therapist has prescribed an individualized exercise program. This program includes 3 days a week (30 minutes each session) of strength- and balance-training exercises. Manuel uses ankle weights for lower body muscle-strengthening exercises and does a series of balance exercises. He does this program with the assistance of a residential aide.

- Manuel's residence includes a garden with walking paths and benches. He has gradually increased his physical activity to walking about 10 minutes each day. On some days he can walk more than on others, but he tries to walk a little every day. The plan is for him to sustain this level of activity for several weeks.

- After he builds strength and his balance improves, Manuel will consider increasing his level of activity and joining an exercise class specially designed to reduce the risk of falls in older people.

Anthony: A 65-Year-Old Man Living in a Retirement Community

Anthony has been active and fit all his life. He does 180 minutes of relatively vigorous-intensity activity each week, plus muscle-strengthening activities on 3 days.

- Six days a week, Anthony gets up early and runs 3 miles, which takes about 30 minutes.

- With help from staff at his community's fitness facility, Anthony designed a weight-lifting program using weight machines. He does this program on 3 days.

Safe and Active

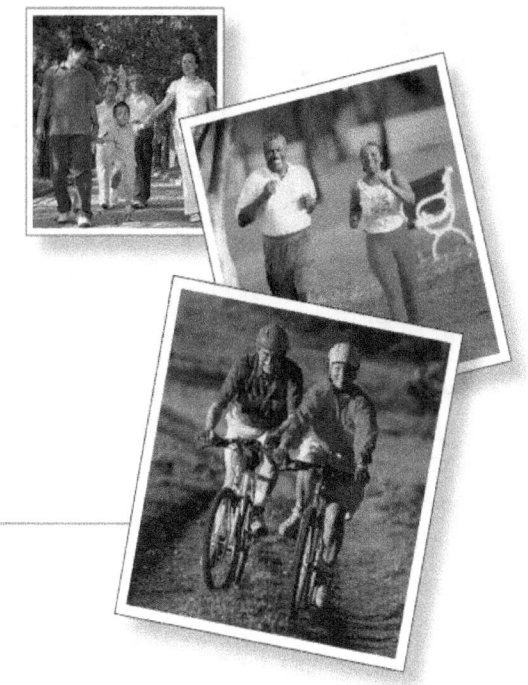

Although physical activity has many health benefits, injuries and other adverse events do sometimes happen. The most common injuries affect the musculoskeletal system (the bones, joints, muscles, ligaments, and tendons). Other adverse events can also occur during activity, such as overheating and dehydration. On rare occasions, people have heart attacks during activity.

The good news is that scientific evidence strongly shows that physical activity is safe for almost everyone. Moreover, the health benefits of physical activity far outweigh the risks.

Still, people may hesitate to become physically active because of concern they'll get hurt. For these people, there is even more good news: They can take steps that are proven to reduce their risk of injury and adverse events.

The Guidelines in this chapter provide advice to help people do physical activity safely. Most advice applies to people of all ages. Specific guidance for particular age groups and people with certain conditions is also provided.

Explaining the Guidelines

Physical Activity Is Safe for Almost Everyone

Most people are not likely to be injured when doing moderate-intensity activities in amounts that meet the *Physical Activity Guidelines*. However, injuries and other adverse events do sometimes happen. The most common problems are musculoskeletal injuries. Even so, studies show that only one such injury occurs for every 1,000 hours of walking for exercise, and fewer than four injuries occur for every 1,000 hours of running.

Both physical fitness and total amount of physical activity affect risk of musculoskeletal injuries. People who are physically fit have a lower risk of injury than people who are not. People who do more activity generally have a higher risk of injury than people who do less activity. So what should people do if they want to be active and safe? The best strategies are to:

- Be regularly physically active to increase physical fitness; and

- Follow the other guidance in this chapter (especially increasing physical activity gradually over time)

To do physical activity safely and reduce risk of injuries and other adverse events, people should:

- Understand the risks and yet be confident that physical activity is safe for almost everyone.

- Choose to do types of physical activity that are appropriate for their current fitness level and health goals, because some activities are safer than others.

- Increase physical activity gradually over time whenever more activity is necessary to meet guidelines or health goals. Inactive people should "start low and go slow" by gradually increasing how often and how long activities are done.

- Protect themselves by using appropriate gear and sports equipment, looking for safe environments, following rules and policies, and making sensible choices about when, where, and how to be active.

- Be under the care of a health-care provider if they have chronic conditions or symptoms. People with chronic conditions and symptoms should consult their health-care provider about the types and amounts of activity appropriate for them.

to minimize the injury risk from doing medium to high amounts of activity.

Following these strategies may reduce *overall* injury risk. Active people are more likely to have an activity-related injury than inactive people. But they appear less likely to have non-activity-related injuries, such as work-related injuries or injuries that occur around the home or from motor vehicle crashes.

Choose Appropriate Types and Amounts of Activity

People can reduce their risk of injury by choosing appropriate types of activity. As the table shows, the safest activities are moderate intensity and low impact, and don't involve purposeful collision or contact.

Walking for exercise, gardening or yard work, bicycling or exercise cycling, dancing, swimming, and golf are activities with the lowest injury rates. In the amounts commonly done by adults, walking (a moderate-intensity and low-impact activity) has a third or less of the injury risk of running (a vigorous-intensity and higher impact activity).

The risk of injury for a type of physical activity can also differ according to the purpose of the activity. For example, recreational bicycling or bicycling for

The Continuum of Injury Risk Associated With Different Types of Activity

Injury Risk Level	Activity Type	Examples
Lower Risk	Commuting	Walking, bicycling
	Lifestyle	Home repair, gardening/ yard work
	Recreation/sports No contact	Walking for exercise, golf, dancing, swimming, running, tennis
	Recreation/sports Limited contact	Bicycling, aerobics, skiing, volleyball, baseball, softball
Higher Risk	Recreation/sports Collision/contact	Football, hockey, soccer, basketball

Note: The same activity done for different purposes and with different frequency, intensity, and duration leads to different injury rates. Competitive activities tend to have higher injury rates than non-competitive activities, likely due to different degrees of intensity of participation.

transportation leads to fewer injuries than training for and competing in bicycle races.

People who have had a past injury are at risk of injuring that body part again. The risk of injury can be reduced by performing appropriate amounts of activity and setting appropriate personal goals. Performing a

The risk of injury

to bones, muscles, and joints is directly related to the gap between a person's usual level of activity and a new level of activity.

variety of different physical activities may also reduce the risk of overuse injury.

Increase Physical Activity Gradually Over Time

Scientific studies indicate that the risk of injury to bones, muscles, and joints is directly related to the gap between a person's usual level of activity and a new level of activity. The size of this gap is called the amount of overload. Creating a small overload and waiting for the body to adapt and recover reduces the risk of injury. When amounts of physical activity need to be increased to meet the Guidelines or personal goals, physical activity should be increased gradually over time, no matter what the person's current level of physical activity.

Scientists have not established a standard for how to gradually increase physical activity over time. The following recommendations give general guidance for inactive people and those with low levels of physical activity on how to increase physical activity:

- Use relative intensity (intensity of the activity relative to a person's fitness) to guide the level of effort for aerobic activity.

- Generally start with relatively moderate-intensity aerobic activity. Avoid relatively vigorous-intensity activity, such as shoveling snow or running. Adults with a low level of fitness may need to start with light activity, or a mix of light- to moderate-intensity activity.

- First, increase the number of minutes per session (duration), and the number of days per week (frequency) of moderate-intensity activity. Later, if desired, increase the intensity.

- Pay attention to the relative size of the increase in physical activity each week, as this is related to injury risk. For example, a 20-minute increase each week is safer for a person who does 200 minutes a week

of walking (a 10 percent increase), than for a person who does 40 minutes a week (a 50 percent increase).

The available scientific evidence suggests that adding a small and comfortable amount of light- to moderate-intensity activity, such as 5 to15 minutes of walking per session, 2 to 3 times a week, to one's usual activities has a low risk of musculoskeletal injury and no known risk of severe cardiac events. Because this range is rather wide, people should consider three factors in individualizing their rate of increase: age, level of fitness, and prior experience.

Age

The amount of time required to adapt to a new level of activity probably depends on age. Youth and young adults probably can safely increase activity by small amounts every week or 2. Older adults appear to require more time to adapt to a new level of activity, in the range of 2 to 4 weeks.

Level of Fitness

Less fit adults are at higher risk of injury when doing a given amount of activity, compared to fitter adults. Slower rates of increase over time may reduce injury risk. This guidance applies to overweight and obese adults, as they are commonly less physically fit.

Prior Experience

People can use their experience to learn to increase physical activity over time in ways that minimize the risk of overuse injury. Generally, if an overuse injury occurred in the past with a certain rate of progression, a person should increase activity more slowly the next time.

Take Appropriate Precautions

Taking appropriate precautions means using the right gear and equipment, choosing safe environments in which to be active, following rules and policies, and making sensible choices about how, when, and where to be active.

Use Protective Gear and Appropriate Equipment
Using personal protective gear can reduce the frequency of injury. Personal protective gear is something worn by a person to protect a specific body part. Examples include helmets, eyewear and goggles, shin guards, elbow and knee pads, and mouth guards.

Using appropriate sports equipment can also reduce risk of injury. Sports equipment refers to sport or activity-specific tools, such as balls, bats, sticks, and shoes.

For the most benefit, protective equipment and gear should be:

- The right equipment for the activity;

- Appropriately fitted;

- Appropriately maintained; and

- Used consistently and correctly.

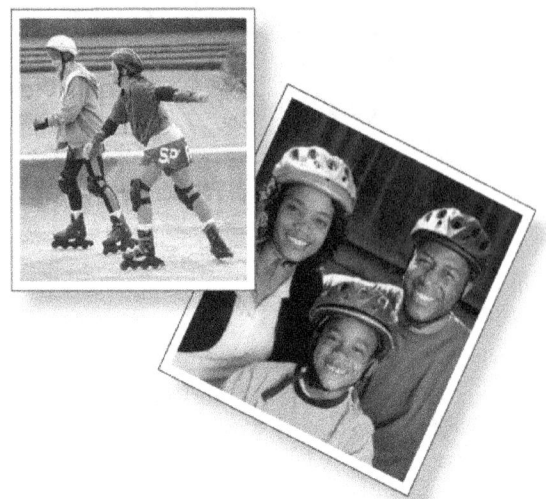

For More Information

See Appendix 2 for a resource chart that provides selected examples of injury prevention strategies for common physical activities.

Be Active in Safe Environments
People can reduce their injury risks by paying attention to the places they choose to be active. To help themselves stay safe, people can look for:

- Physical separation from motor vehicles, such as sidewalks, walking paths, or bike lanes;

- Neighborhoods with traffic-calming measures that slow down traffic;

- Places to be active that are well-lighted, where other people are present, and that are well-maintained (no litter, broken windows);

- Shock-absorbing surfaces on playgrounds;

- Well-maintained playing fields and courts without holes or obstacles;

- Breakaway bases at baseball and softball fields; and

- Padded and anchored goals and goal posts at soccer and football fields.

Follow Rules and Policies That Promote Safety
Rules, policies, legislation, and laws are potentially the most effective and wide-reaching way to reduce activity-related injuries. To get the benefit, individuals should look for and follow these rules, policies, and laws. For example, policies that promote the use of bicycle helmets reduce the risk of head injury among cyclists. Rules against diving into shallow water at swimming pools prevent head and neck injuries.

Make Sensible Choices About How, When, and Where To Be Active
A person's choices can obviously influence the risk of adverse events. By making sensible choices, injuries and adverse events can be prevented. Consider weather conditions, such as extremes of heat and cold. For example, during very hot and humid weather, people lessen the chances of dehydration and heat stress by:

- Exercising in the cool of early morning as opposed to mid-day heat;

- Switching to indoor activities (playing basketball in the gym rather than on the playground);

- Changing the type of activity (swimming rather than playing soccer);

Inactive people

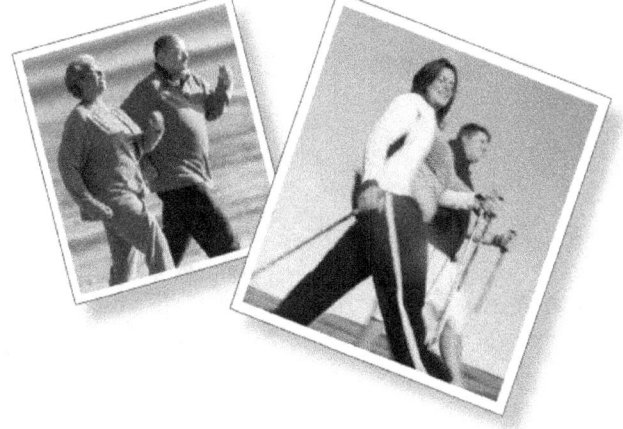

who gradually progress over time to relatively moderate-intensity activity have no known risk of sudden cardiac events, and very low risk of bone, muscle, or joint injuries.

- Lowering the intensity of activity (walking rather than running); and

- Paying close attention to rest, shade, drinking enough fluids, and other ways to minimize effects of heat.

Exposure to air pollution is associated with several adverse health outcomes, including asthma attacks and abnormal heart rhythms. People who can modify the location or time of exercise may wish to reduce these risks by exercising away from heavy traffic and industrial sites, especially during rush hour or times when pollution is known to be high. However, current evidence indicates that the benefits of being active, even in polluted air, outweigh the risk of being inactive.

Advice From Health-Care Providers

The protective value of a medical consultation for persons with or without chronic diseases who are interested in increasing their physical activity level is not established. People without diagnosed chronic conditions (such as diabetes, heart disease, or osteoarthritis) and who do not have symptoms (such as chest pain or pressure, dizziness, or joint pain) do not need to consult a health-care provider about physical activity.

Inactive people who gradually progress over time to relatively moderate-intensity activity have no known risk of sudden cardiac events, and very low risk of bone, muscle, or joint injuries. A person who is habitually active with moderate-intensity activity can gradually increase to vigorous intensity without needing to consult a health-care provider. People who

develop new symptoms when increasing their levels of activity should consult a health-care provider.

Health-care providers can provide useful personalized advice on how to reduce risk of injuries. For people who wish to seek the advice of a health-care provider, it is particularly appropriate to do so when contemplating vigorous-intensity activity, because the risks of this activity are higher than the risks of moderate-intensity activity.

For More Information

See Chapter 4—Active Adults, for guidance and examples of how to gradually increase activity levels.

The choice of appropriate types and amounts of physical activity can be affected by chronic conditions. People with symptoms or known chronic conditions should be under the regular care of a health-care provider. In consultation with their provider, they can develop a physical activity plan that is appropriate for them. People with chronic conditions typically find that moderate-intensity activity is safe and beneficial. However, they may need to take special precautions. For example, people with diabetes need to pay special attention to blood sugar control and proper footwear during activity.

Women who are pregnant and those who've recently had a baby should be under the regular care of a health-care provider. Moderate-intensity physical activity is generally safe for women with uncomplicated pregnancies, but women should talk with their provider about how to adjust the amounts and types of activity while they are pregnant and right after the baby's birth.

During pregnancy, women should avoid:

For More Information

See Chapter 7—Additional Considerations for Some Adults, for more details about physical activity during pregnancy and the postpartum period.

- Doing activities that involve lying on their back after the first trimester of pregnancy; and

- Doing activities with high risk of falling or abdominal trauma, including contact or collision sports, such as horseback riding, soccer, basketball, and downhill skiing.

Gradually Increasing Physical Activity Over Time: Real-Life Examples

Here are two examples that show how people at different ages, levels of fitness, and levels of experience can safely become more active over time.

Bill: A Man Who Has Been Inactive for Many Years

Bill wants to work his way up to the equivalent of 180 to 210 minutes (3 hours to 3 hours and 30 minutes) of walking a week. On weekdays he has time for up to 45 minutes of walking, and he plans to do something physically active each weekend. He decides to start with walking because it is moderate intensity and has a low risk of injury.

- The first week, Bill starts at a low level. He walks 10 minutes a day 3 days a week. Sometimes he divides the 10 minutes a day into two sessions. He prefers to alternate rest days and active days. (Total = 30 minutes a week.)

- Between weeks 3 and 8, Bill increases duration by adding 5 minutes a day and continues walking on 3 non-consecutive days each week. The weekly increase is 15 minutes. (Week 3 total = 45 minutes. Week 8 total = 120 minutes or 2 hours.)

- In week 9, Bill adds another day of moderate-intensity activity on the weekend, and starts doing a variety of activities, including biking, hiking, and an aerobics class. Gradually increasing the minutes of

activity, by week 12 he is doing 60 minutes or more of moderate-intensity activity on the weekend.

Reaching his goal: Over 3 months, Bill has increased to a total of 180 moderate-intensity minutes a week.

Kim: An Active Woman

Kim currently does 150 minutes (2 hours and 30 minutes) a week of moderate-intensity activity. She wants to work up to at least the equivalent of 300 minutes (5 hours) of moderate-intensity activity a week. She also wants to shift some of that moderate-intensity activity to vigorous-intensity activity. Her current 150 minutes a week includes:

- Thirty minutes of mowing the grass 1 day a week;

- Thirty minutes of brisk walking 4 days a week; and

- Fifteen minutes of muscle-strengthening exercises 2 days a week.

Increasing frequency and duration:

- Over a month, Kim adds walking on another weekday, and she gradually adds 15 minutes of moderate-intensity activity on each of the 5 walking days each week. This provides an additional 105 minutes (1 hour and 45 minutes) of moderate-intensity activity.

Increasing intensity:

- Over the next month, Kim decides to replace some walking with jogging. Instead of walking 45 minutes, she walks for 30 minutes and jogs for 15 minutes on each weekday, providing the equivalent of 300 minutes a week of moderate-intensity physical activity from her walking and jogging.

Reaching her goal: After these increases, Kim is doing a total of 180 minutes of moderate-intensity activity each week (walking and mowing) and also doing 75 minutes (1 hour and 15 minutes) of vigorous-intensity jogging. One minute of vigorous-intensity activity is about the same as 2 minutes of moderate-intensity activity, so she is now doing the equivalent of 330 moderate-intensity minutes (5 hours and 30 minutes) a week. She has more than met her goal.

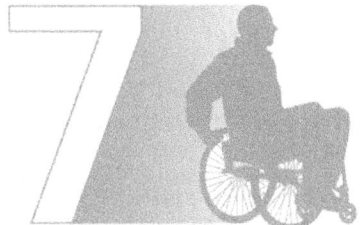

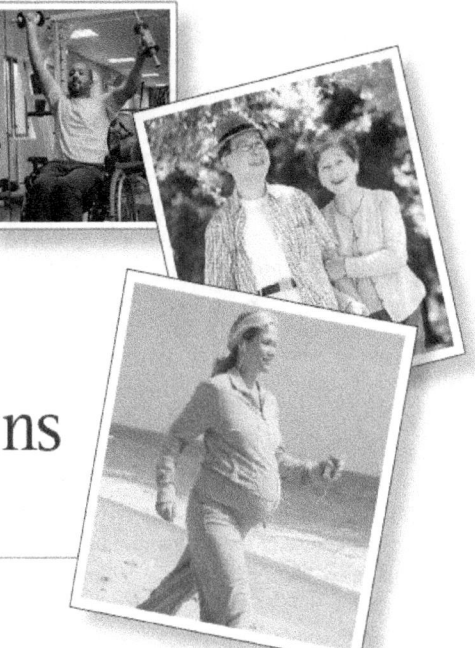

Additional Considerations for Some Adults

All Americans should be physically active to improve overall health and fitness and to prevent many adverse health outcomes. Most Americans should follow the Guidelines of the child and adolescent, adult, or older adult chapters, depending upon their age. However, some people have conditions that raise special issues about recommended types and amounts of physical activity. This chapter provides guidance on physical activity for healthy women who are pregnant and for people with disabilities. This chapter also affirms and illustrates how physical activity is generally appropriate for adults with chronic conditions by considering three groups of adults:

- Adults with osteoarthritis;
- Adults with type 2 diabetes; and
- Adults who are cancer survivors.

Physical Activity for Women During Pregnancy and the Postpartum Period

Physical activity during pregnancy benefits a woman's overall health. For example, moderate-intensity physical activity by healthy women during pregnancy maintains or increases cardiorespiratory fitness.

Strong scientific evidence shows that the risks of moderate-intensity activity done by healthy women during pregnancy are very low, and do not increase risk of low birth weight, preterm delivery, or early pregnancy loss. Some evidence suggests that physical activity reduces the risk of pregnancy complications, such as preeclampsia and gestational diabetes, and reduces the length of labor, but this evidence is not conclusive.

During a normal postpartum period, regular physical activity continues to benefit a woman's overall health. Studies show that moderate-intensity physical activity during the period following the birth of a child increases a woman's cardiorespiratory fitness and improves her mood. Such activity does not appear to have adverse effects on breast milk volume, breast milk composition, or infant growth.

Physical activity also helps women achieve and maintain a healthy weight during the postpartum period, and when combined with caloric restriction, helps promote weight loss.

- Healthy women who are not already highly active or doing vigorous-intensity activity should get at least 150 minutes (2 hours and 30 minutes) of moderate-intensity aerobic activity per week during pregnancy and the postpartum period. Preferably, this activity should be spread throughout the week.

- Pregnant women who habitually engage in vigorous-intensity aerobic activity or are highly active can continue physical activity during pregnancy and the postpartum period, provided that they remain healthy and discuss with their health-care provider how and when activity should be adjusted over time.

Explaining the Guidelines

Women who are pregnant should be under the care of a health-care provider with whom they can discuss how to adjust amounts of physical activity during pregnancy and the postpartum period. Unless a woman has medical reasons to avoid physical activity during pregnancy, she can begin or continue moderate-intensity aerobic physical activity during her pregnancy and after the baby is born.

When beginning physical activity during pregnancy, women should increase the amount gradually over time. The effects of vigorous-intensity aerobic activity during pregnancy have not been studied carefully, so there is no basis for recommending that women should begin vigorous-intensity activity during pregnancy.

Women who habitually do vigorous-intensity activity or high amounts of activity or strength training should continue to be physically active during pregnancy and after giving birth. They generally do not need to drastically reduce their activity levels, provided that they remain healthy and discuss with their health-care provider how to adjust activity levels during this time.

During pregnancy, women should avoid doing exercises involving lying on their back after the first trimester of pregnancy. They should also avoid doing activities that increase the risk of falling or abdominal trauma, including contact or collision sports, such as horseback riding, downhill skiing, soccer, and basketball.

Physical Activity for People With Disabilities

The benefits of physical activity for people with disabilities have been studied in diverse groups. These groups include stroke victims, people with spinal cord injury, multiple sclerosis, Parkinson's disease, muscular dystrophy, cerebral palsy, traumatic brain injury, limb amputations, mental illness, intellectual disability, and dementia.

Overall, the evidence shows that regular physical activity provides important health benefits for people with disabilities. The benefits include improved cardiovascular and muscle fitness, improved mental health, and better ability to do tasks of daily life. Sufficient evidence now exists to recommend that adults with disabilities should get regular physical activity. Physical activity in children and adolescents with disabilities is considered in Chapter 3—Active Children and Adolescents.

For More Information

See Chapter 2—Physical Activity Has Many Health Benefits, for details.

Explaining the Guidelines

In consultation with their health-care providers, people with disabilities should understand how their disabilities affect their ability to do physical activity. Some may be capable of doing medium to high amounts of physical activity, and they should essentially follow the Guidelines for adults.

For More Information

See Chapter 4—Active Adults, for details on these Guidelines and how to meet them.

Some people with disabilities are not able to follow the Guidelines for adults. These people should adapt their physical activity program to match their abilities, in consultation with their health-care providers. Studies show that physical activity can be done safely when the program is matched to an individual's abilities.

Meeting the Guidelines

People with disabilities are encouraged to get advice from professionals with experience in physical activity and disability because matching activity to abilities can require modifying physical activity in many different ways. Some people with disabilities also need help with their exercise program. For example, some people may need supervision when performing muscle-strengthening activities, such as lifting weights.

Physical Activity for People With Chronic Medical Conditions

Adults with chronic conditions should engage in regular physical activity because it can help promote their quality of life and reduce the risk of developing new conditions. The type and amount of physical activity should be determined by a person's abilities and the severity of the chronic condition. Three examples are provided below to illustrate the benefits of physical activity for persons with chronic conditions.

For many chronic conditions, physical activity provides therapeutic benefits and is part of recommended treatment for the condition. However, this chapter does not discuss therapeutic exercise or rehabilitation.

Example 1. Physical Activity for Adults With Osteoarthritis

Osteoarthritis is a common condition in older adults, and people can live many years with osteoarthritis. People with osteoarthritis are commonly concerned that physical activity can make their condition worse. Osteoarthritis can be painful and cause fatigue, making it hard to begin or maintain regular physical activity. Yet people with this condition should get regular physical activity to lower their risk of getting other chronic diseases, such as heart disease or type 2 diabetes, and to help maintain a healthy body weight.

For More Information

See Chapter 2—Physical Activity Has Many Health Benefits, for details on these benefits.

Strong scientific evidence indicates that both aerobic activity and muscle-strengthening activity provide therapeutic benefits for persons with osteoarthritis. When done safely, physical activity does not make the disease or the pain worse. Studies show that adults with osteoarthritis can expect improvements in pain, physical function, quality of life, and mental health with regular physical activity.

People with osteoarthritis should match the type and amount of physical activity to their abilities and the severity of their condition. Most people can usually do

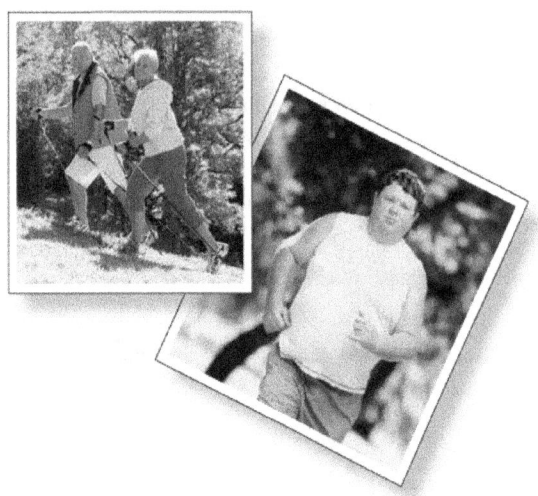

For example, strong scientific evidence shows that physical activity protects against heart disease in people with diabetes. Moderate-intensity activity for about 150 minutes a week helps to substantially lower the risk of heart disease. A person who moves toward 300 minutes (5 hours) or more of moderate-intensity activity a week gets even greater benefit.

Adults with chronic conditions should work with their health-care providers to adapt physical activity so that it is appropriate for their condition. For example, people with diabetes must be careful to monitor their blood glucose and avoid injury to their feet.

Example 3. Physical Activity for Cancer Survivors

With modern treatments, many people with cancer can either be cured or survive for many years, living long enough to be at risk of other chronic conditions, such as high blood pressure or type 2 diabetes. Some cancer survivors are at risk of recurrence of the original cancer. Some have experienced side effects of the cancer treatment.

Like other adults, cancer survivors should engage in regular physical activity for its preventive benefits. Physical activity in cancer survivors can reduce risk of new chronic diseases. Further, studies suggest physically active adults with breast or colon cancer are less like to die prematurely or have a recurrence of the cancer. Physical activity may also play a role in reducing adverse effects of cancer treatment.

Cancer survivors, like other adults with chronic conditions, should consult their health-care providers to match their physical activity plan to their abilities and health status.

moderate-intensity activity for 150 minutes (2 hours and 30 minutes) a week or more, and may choose to be active 3 to 5 days a week for 30 to 60 minutes per episode. Some people with arthritis can safely do more than 150 minutes of moderate-intensity activity each week and may be able to tolerate equivalent amounts of vigorous-intensity activity. Health-care providers typically counsel people with osteoarthritis to do activities that are low impact, not painful, and have low risk of joint injury. Swimming, walking, and strength-training are good examples of this type of activity.

Example 2. Physical Activity for Adults With Type 2 Diabetes

Physical activity in adults with type 2 diabetes shows how important it can be for people with a chronic disease to be active. Physical activity has important therapeutic effects in people with diabetes, but it is also routinely recommended to reduce risk of other diseases and help promote a healthy body weight.

Key Messages for People With Chronic Medical Conditions

- Adults with chronic conditions obtain important health benefits from regular physical activity.

- When adults with chronic conditions do activity according to their abilities, physical activity is safe.

- Adults with chronic conditions should be under the care of health-care providers. People with chronic conditions and symptoms should consult their health-care providers about the types and amounts of activity appropriate for them.

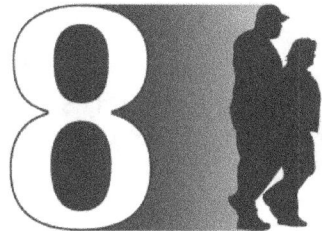

Taking Action: Increasing Physical Activity Levels of Americans

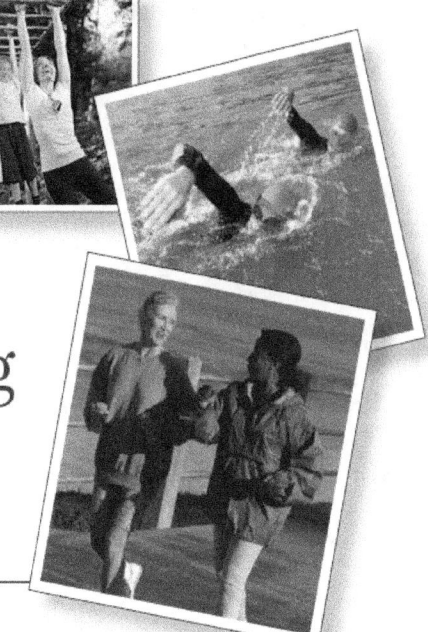

The low level of physical activity among Americans is a major contributor to the burden of chronic disease. This burden is costly in terms of quality of life and economic resources needed to provide medical care. Like life in other modern societies around the world, life in the United States requires very little daily physical activity. The amount of physical activity we do is largely a matter of personal choice and the environmental conditions under which we live. So far, little progress has been made in meeting our national health objectives for physical activity.

Based on a careful review of the science, the *Physical Activity Guidelines* provides essential guidance to help Americans achieve the health benefits of regular physical activity. However, providing guidance by itself is not enough to produce change. Action is necessary. Regular physical activity needs to be made the easy choice for Americans.

To accomplish this goal, public health research suggests the use of a "socio-ecologic" approach. This comprehensive approach involves action at all levels of society: individual, interpersonal, organizational, community, and public policy. Example actions include:

- Personal goal setting (individual level);

- Social support and encouragement to be active (interpersonal level);

- Promotion of physical activity as part of worksite health promotion programs (organizational);

- Good access to parks and recreational facilities in neighborhoods (community); and

- Promotion of policies that support families who want their children to walk or bike to school (public policy).

For More Information

See Appendix 3—Federal Web Sites That Promote Physical Activity, for useful resources at all these levels.

To give a sense of how to make regular physical activity the easy choice, the remainder of this chapter first considers steps individuals can take to adopt an active lifestyle. Then it considers steps society can take to support and facilitate active lifestyles. The purpose is to illustrate achievable steps that will make a difference, not to address everything that needs to be done.

What Can Adults Do To Get Enough Physical Activity?

Adults can find advice on how to be active from many sources, including fitness professionals, health-care providers, books, and Web sites. Here are three commonly cited steps adults can take to help meet the Guidelines.

Personalize the Benefits of Regular Physical Activity

Adults need to identify benefits of personal value to them. For many people, the health benefits, which are the focus of the *Physical Activity Guidelines for Americans,* are compelling enough. For others, different reasons are key motivators to be active. For example, physical activity:

- Provides opportunities to enjoy recreational activities, often in a social setting;

- Improves personal appearance;

- Provides a chance to help a spouse lose weight;

- Improves the quality of sleep;

- Reduces feelings of low energy; and

- Gives older adults a greater opportunity to live independently in the community.

Set Personal Goals for Physical Activity

The Guidelines alone don't provide enough information for individuals to decide the types and amounts of activity that are appropriate for them. Individuals should set goals for activity that allow them to achieve benefits they value. Simple goals are fine. For example, a brisk walk in the neighborhood with friends for 45 minutes 3 days a week and walking to lunch twice a week may be just the right approach for someone who wants to increase both physical activity and social opportunities.

In setting goals, people can consider doing a variety of activities and try both indoor and outdoor activities. In particular, public parks and recreation areas in the United States offer opportunities to experience nature and be physically active at the same time.

The best

physical activity is the one that is enjoyable enough to do regularly.

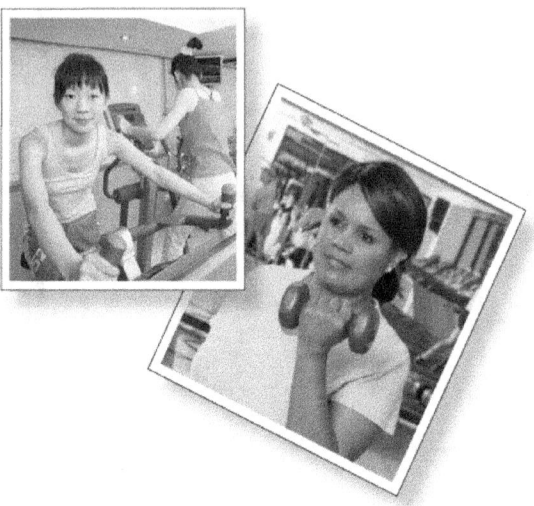

Develop Knowledge To Attain Goals

It is important to learn about the types and amount of activity needed to attain personal goals. For example, if weight loss is a goal, it's useful to know that vigorous-intensity activity can be much more time-efficient in burning calories than moderate-intensity activity. If running is a goal, it's important to learn how to reduce risk of running injuries by selecting an appropriate training program and proper shoes. If regular walking is a goal, learning about neighborhood walking trails can help a person attain the goal.

How Can We Help Children and Adolescents Get Enough Physical Activity?

Many children and adolescents are naturally physically active, and they need opportunities to be active and to learn skills. They benefit from encouragement from parents and other adults. Adults can promote age-appropriate activity in youth through these steps:

- **Provide time for both structured and unstructured physical activity during school and outside of school.** Children need time for active play. Through recess,

Using a Pedometer To Track Walking

For adults who prefer walking as a form of aerobic activity, pedometers or step counters are useful in tracking progress toward personal goals. Popular advice, such as walking 10,000 steps a day, is not a Guideline *per se*, but a way people may choose to meet the Guidelines. The key to using a pedometer to meet the Guidelines is to first set a time goal (minutes of walking a day) and then calculate how many steps are needed each day to reach that goal.

Episodes of brisk walking that last at least 10 minutes count toward meeting the Guidelines. However, just counting steps using a pedometer doesn't ensure that a person will achieve those 10-minute episodes. People generally need to plan episodes of walking if they are to use a pedometer and step goals appropriately.

As a basis for setting step goals, it's preferable that people know how many steps they take per minute of a brisk walk. A person with a low fitness level, who takes fewer steps per minute than a fit adult, will need fewer steps to achieve the same amount of walking time.

One way to set a step goal is the following:

1. To determine usual daily steps from baseline activity, a person wears a pedometer to observe the number of steps taken on several ordinary days with no episodes of walking for exercise. Suppose the average is about 5,000 steps a day.

2. While wearing the pedometer, the person measures the number of steps taken during 10 minutes of an exercise walk. Suppose this is 1,000 steps. Then, for a goal of 40 minutes of walking for exercise, the total number of steps would be 4,000 (1,000 × 4).

3. To calculate a daily step goal, add the usual daily steps (5,000) to the steps required for a 40-minute walk (4,000), to get the total steps per day (5,000 + 4,000 = 9,000).

Each week the person gradually increases the time walking for exercise until the step goal is reached. Rate of progression should be individualized. Some people who start out at 5,000 steps a day can add 500 steps per day each week. Others, who are less fit and starting out at a lower number of steps, should add a smaller number of steps each week.

physical activity breaks, physical education classes, after-school programs, and active time with family and friends, youth can learn about physical activity and spend time doing it.

- **Provide children and adolescents with positive feedback and good role models.** It has been said that if you do not practice what you teach, you are teaching something else. Parents and teachers should model and encourage an active lifestyle for children. Praise, rewards, and encouragement help children to be active. Using physical activity as punishment does not help children to be active.

- **Help young people learn skills required to do physical activity safely.** As appropriate for their age, youth need to understand how to regulate the intensity of activity, increase physical activity gradually over time, set goals, use protective gear and proper equipment, follow rules, and avoid injuries.

- **Promote activities that set the basis for a lifetime of activity.** Children and adolescents should be exposed to a variety of activities, including active recreation, team sports, and individual sports. In this way, they can find activities they can do well and

Communities

can provide many opportunities for physical activity, such as walking trails, bicycle lanes on roads, sidewalks, and sports fields.

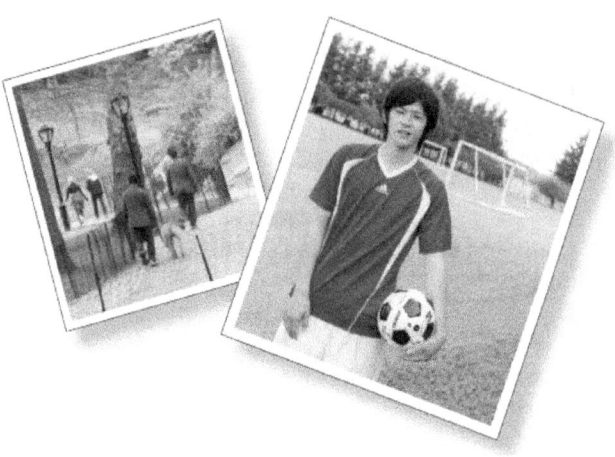

enjoy. Include exposure to activities that adults commonly do, such as jogging, bicycling, hiking, and swimming. Young people should experience non-competitive activities and activities that do not require above-average athletic skills.

What Can Communities Do To Help People Be Active?

Actions by communities can influence whether regular physical activity is an easy choice. Communities can provide many opportunities for physical activity, such as walking trails, bicycle lanes on roads, sidewalks, and sports fields. Organizations in the community have a role to play as well. Schools, places of worship, worksites, and community centers can provide opportunities and encouragement for physical activity.

Use Evidence-Based Approaches and Tailor Them to the Needs of Individual Communities

To be effective, physical activity promotion efforts should use an "evidence-based" approach. The CDC's *Guide to Community Preventive Services*[1] has reviewed many community-level approaches to promote physical activity, including these five strongly recommended strategies:

- **Community-wide campaigns** that combine physical activity messaging (distributed through television, newspapers, radio, and other media) with activities such as physical activity counseling, community health fairs, and the development of walking trails.

- **Physical education classes** to increase activity. Physical education classes should use a curriculum that increases the amount of time students are active during class.

- **Approaches that increase the reach of individual-level interventions.** For example, evidence-based, individual-level interventions can reach more people when they are delivered in group settings.

- **Interventions that increase social support** for physical activity. These interventions start or enhance social-support networks, and include efforts such as organizing a buddy system (two or more people who set regular times to do physical activity together), walking groups, and community dances.

- **Programs to create or enhance access** to places to be physically active. This can include building walking trails and providing public access to school gymnasiums, playgrounds, or community centers. This also includes worksite activity programs that provide access to onsite or offsite fitness rooms, walking breaks, or other opportunities to engage in physical activity. Interventions to improve access should also include outreach that increases awareness of the opportunity to be active.

Involve Many Sectors in Promoting Physical Activity

Implementing community-level approaches to physical activity requires collaboration across sectors.

---

[1]Centers for Disease Control and Prevention. (Last updated February 21, 2008). Physical Activity. In Guide to Community Preventive Services Web site. Retrieved April 17, 2008, from www.thecommunityguide.org/pa.

Implementing

community-level approaches to physical activity requires collaboration across sectors.

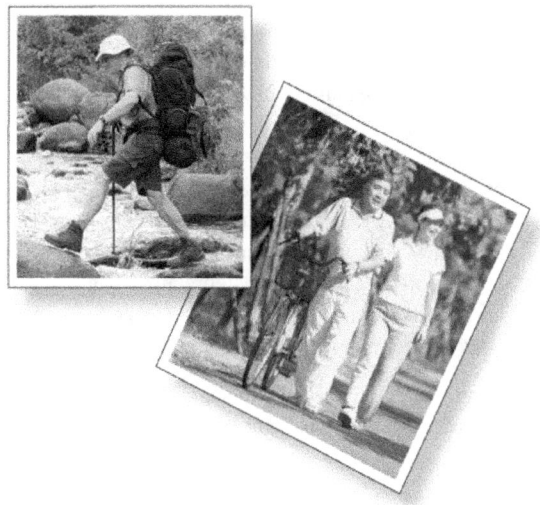

The following list identifies relevant sectors and illustrates roles they play in promoting physical activity. The division of functions in the community into the following sectors does not use mutually exclusive categories. These sectors were chosen simply to illustrate how parts of the community have a role to play in promoting physical activity. Some communities may use different names and divisions of functions.

- **Parks and recreation.** This sector plays a lead role in providing access to places for active recreation, such as playgrounds, hiking and biking trails, basketball courts, sports fields, and swimming pools.

- **Law enforcement.** Concern about crime can deter people from outdoors recreation. Law enforcement can promote a safe environment that facilitates outdoor activity.

- **Urban planning.** Urban planners have a lead role in implementing design principles to promote physical activity.

- **Transportation.** The transportation sector has a lead role in designing and implementing options that provide areas for safe walking and bicycling. Mass transit systems also promote walking, as people

typically walk to and from transit stops. Programs that support safe walking and bicycling to school help children be physically active.

- **Education.** The education sector takes a lead role in providing physical education, after-school sports, and public access to school facilities during after-school hours.

- **Architecture.** Architects and builders can design and construct buildings with active options, such as access to stairs. Campuses should allow pedestrians pleasant and efficient methods of walking within and between buildings.

- **Employers and private organizations.** Employers can encourage workers to be physically active, facilitate active transportation by supplying showers and secure bicycle storage, and provide other incentives to be active. Private and faith-based organizations can support community physical activity initiatives financially or by providing space for programs. Health and fitness facilities and community programs can provide access to exercise programs and equipment for a broad range of people, including older adults and people with disabilities. Local sports organizations can organize road races and events for the public. Senior centers can provide exercise programs for older adults.

- **Health care.** Health-care providers can assess, counsel, and advise patients on physical activity and how to do it safely. Health-care providers can model healthy behaviors by being physically active themselves.

- **Public health.** Public health departments can monitor community progress in providing places and opportunities to be physically active and can track changes in the proportion of the population meeting the *Physical Activity Guidelines for Americans.* They can also take the lead in setting objectives and coordinating activities among sectors. Public health departments and organizations can disseminate appropriate messages and information to the public about physical activity.

Glossary

This section provides definitions for many terms important to physical activity and health. It has been adapted from the glossary provided in the *Physical Activity Guidelines Advisory Committee Report* (http://www.health.gov/PAGuidelines/Report/Default.aspx). It is not meant to be an exhaustive list, and definitions of additional terms can be found in the Committee's report.

Absolute intensity. See **Intensity.**

Accumulate. The concept of meeting a specific physical activity dose or goal by performing activity in short bouts, then adding together the time spent during each of these bouts. For example, a goal of 30 minutes a day could be met by performing 3 bouts of 10 minutes each throughout the day.

Adaptation. The body's response to exercise or activity. Some of the body's structures and functions favorably adjust to the increase in demands placed on them whenever physical activity of a greater amount or higher intensity is performed than what is usual for the individual. These adaptations are the basis for much of the improved health and fitness associated with increases in physical activity.

Adverse event. In the context of physical activity, a negative health event. Examples of adverse events as a result of physical activity include musculoskeletal injuries (injury to bone, muscles, or joints), heat-related conditions (heat exhaustion), and cardiovascular (heart attack or stroke) events.

Aerobic capacity. See **Maximal oxygen uptake.**

Aerobic physical activity. Activity in which the body's large muscles move in a rhythmic manner for a sustained period of time. Aerobic activity, also called endurance activity, improves cardiorespiratory fitness. Examples include walking, running, and swimming, and bicycling.

Balance. A performance-related component of physical fitness that involves the maintenance of the body's equilibrium while stationary or moving.

Balance training. Static and dynamic exercises that are designed to improve individuals' ability to withstand challenges from postural sway or destabilizing stimuli caused by self-motion, the environment, or other objects.

Baseline activity. The light-intensity activities of daily life, such as standing, walking slowly, and lifting lightweight objects. People who do only baseline activity are considered to be inactive.

Body composition. A health-related component of physical fitness that applies to body weight and the relative amounts of muscle, fat, bone, and other vital tissues of the body. Most often, the components are limited to fat and lean body mass (or fat-free mass).

Bone-strengthening activity. Physical activity primarily designed to increase the strength of specific sites in bones that make up the skeletal system. Bone-strengthening activities produce an impact or tension force on the bones that promotes bone growth and strength. Running, jumping rope, and lifting weights are examples of bone-strengthening activities.

Cardiorespiratory fitness (endurance). A health-related component of physical fitness that is the ability of the circulatory and respiratory systems to supply oxygen during sustained physical activity. Cardiorespiratory fitness is usually expressed as measured or estimated maximal oxygen uptake (VO_2max). See **Maximal oxygen uptake.**

Dose response. The relation between the dose of physical activity and the health or fitness outcome of interest. In the field of physical activity, "dose" refers to the amount of physical activity performed by the subject or participants. The total dose, or amount, is determined by the three components of activity: frequency, duration, and intensity.

Duration. The length of time in which an activity or exercise is performed. Duration is generally expressed in minutes.

Endurance activity. See **Aerobic physical activity.**

Exercise. A subcategory of physical activity that is planned, structured, repetitive, and purposive in the sense that the improvement or maintenance of one or more components of physical fitness is the objective. "Exercise" and "exercise training" frequently are used interchangeably and generally refer to physical activity performed during leisure time with the primary purpose of improving or maintaining physical fitness, physical performance, or health.

Fitness. See **Physical fitness.**

Flexibility. A health- and performance-related component of physical fitness that is the range of motion possible at a joint. Flexibility is specific to each joint and depends on a number of specific variables, including but not limited to the tightness of specific ligaments and tendons. Flexibility exercises enhance the ability of a joint to move through its full range of motion.

Frequency. The number of times an exercise or activity is performed. Frequency is generally expressed in sessions, episodes, or bouts per week.

Health. A human condition with physical, social and psychological dimensions, each characterized on a continuum with positive and negative poles. Positive health is associated with a capacity to enjoy life and to withstand challenges; it is not merely the absence of disease. Negative health is associated with illness, and in the extreme, with premature death.

Health-enhancing physical activity. Activity that, when added to baseline activity, produces health benefits. Brisk walking, jumping rope, dancing, playing tennis or soccer, lifting weights, climbing on playground equipment at recess, and doing yoga are all examples of health-enhancing physical activity.

Health-related fitness. A type of physical fitness that includes cardiorespiratory fitness, muscular strength and endurance, body composition, flexibility, and balance.

Intensity. Intensity refers to how much work is being performed or the magnitude of the effort required to perform an activity or exercise. Intensity can be expressed either in *absolute* or *relative* terms.

- **Absolute.** The absolute intensity of an activity is determined by the rate of work being performed and does not take into account the physiologic capacity of the individual. For aerobic activity, absolute intensity typically is expressed as the rate of energy expenditure (for example, milliliters per kilogram per minute of oxygen being consumed, kilocalories per minute, or METs) or, for some activities, simply as the speed of the activity (for example, walking at 3 miles an hour, jogging at 6 miles an hour), or physiologic response to the intensity (for example, heart rate). For resistance activity or exercise, intensity frequently is expressed as the amount of weight lifted or moved.

- **Relative.** Relative intensity takes into account or adjusts for a person's exercise capacity. For aerobic exercise, relative intensity is expressed as a percent of a person's aerobic capacity (VO_2max) or VO_2 reserve, or as a percent of a person's measured or estimated maximum heart rate (heart rate reserve). It also can be expressed as an index of how hard the person feels he or she is exercising (for example, a 0 to 10 scale).

Lifestyle activities. This term is frequently used to encompass activities that a person carries out in the course of daily life and that can contribute to sizeable energy expenditure. Examples include taking the stairs instead of using the elevator, walking to do errands instead of driving, getting off a bus one stop early, or parking farther away than usual to walk to a destination.

Maximal oxygen uptake (VO_2max). The body's capacity to transport and use oxygen during a maximal exertion involving dynamic contraction of large muscle groups, such as during running or cycling. Also known as maximal aerobic power and cardiorespiratory endurance capacity.

MET. MET refers to metabolic equivalent, and 1 MET is the rate of energy expenditure while sitting at rest. It is taken by convention to be an oxygen uptake of 3.5 milliliters per kilogram of body weight per minute. Physical activities frequently are classified by their intensity using the MET as a reference.

Moderate-intensity physical activity. On an absolute scale, physical activity that is done at 3.0 to 5.9 times the intensity of rest. On a scale relative to an individual's personal capacity, moderate-intensity physical activity is usually a 5 or 6 on a scale of 0 to 10.

Muscle-strengthening activity (strength training, resistance training, or muscular strength and endurance exercises). Physical activity, including exercise, that increases skeletal muscle strength, power, endurance, and mass.

Overload. The amount of new activity added to a person's usual level of activity. The risk of injury to bones, muscles, and joints is directly related to the size of the gap between these two levels. This gap is called the amount of overload.

Performance-related fitness. Those attributes that significantly contribute to athletic performance, including aerobic endurance or power, muscle strength and power, speed of movement, and reaction time.

Physical activity. Any bodily movement produced by the contraction of skeletal muscle that increases energy expenditure above a basal level. In these Guidelines, physical activity generally refers to the subset of physical activity that enhances health.

Physical fitness. The ability to carry out daily tasks with vigor and alertness, without undue fatigue, and with ample energy to enjoy leisure-time pursuits and respond to emergencies. Physical fitness includes a number of components consisting of cardiorespiratory endurance (aerobic power), skeletal muscle endurance, skeletal muscle strength, skeletal muscle power, flexibility, balance, speed of movement, reaction time, and body composition.

Progression. The process of increasing the intensity, duration, frequency, or amount of activity or exercise as the body adapts to a given activity pattern.

Relative intensity. See **Intensity.**

Relative risk. The risk of a (typically) adverse health outcome among a group of people with a certain condition compared to a group of people without the condition. In physical activity, relative risk is typically the ratio of the risk of a disease or disorder when comparing groups of people who vary in their amount of physical activity.

Repetitions. The number of times a person lifts a weight in muscle-strengthening activities. Repetitions are analogous to duration in aerobic activity.

Resistance training. See **Muscle-strengthening activity.**

Specificity. A principle of exercise physiology that indicates that physiologic changes in the human body in response to physical activity are highly dependent on the type of physical activity. For example, the physiologic effects of walking are largely specific to the lower body and the cardiovascular system.

Strength. A health and performance component of physical fitness that is the ability of a muscle or muscle group to exert force.

Strength training. See **Muscle-strengthening activity.**

Vigorous-intensity physical activity. On an absolute scale, physical activity that is done at 6.0 or more times the intensity of rest. On a scale relative to an individual's personal capacity, vigorous-intensity physical activity is usually a 7 or 8 on a scale of 0 to 10.

Appendix 1. Translating Scientific Evidence About Total Amount and Intensity of Physical Activity Into Guidelines

This appendix discusses two issues that arise when translating scientific evidence into physical activity guidance for the public:

- In scientific terms, total weekly physical activity in the range of 500 to 1,000 MET-minutes produces substantial health benefits for adults. How should this finding be simplified and translated into Guidelines that are understandable by the public?

- Two methods are used to assess the intensity of aerobic physical activity, termed "absolute intensity" and "relative intensity." Should the Guidelines specify one method or allow both?

After discussing background information related to these questions, this appendix explains the approach taken on these two issues in the *Physical Activity Guidelines for Americans*.

Background

The Guidelines are derived from an evidence-based report on the health benefits of physical activity, written by the Physical Activity Guidelines Advisory Committee. As background, this appendix first briefly explains the concept of METs and MET-minutes. It then discusses three key findings of the Advisory Committee report, and finally discusses the difference between absolute and relative intensity.

For More Information

See Chapter 1—Introducing the *2008 Physical Activity Guidelines for Americans*, for details on the Advisory Committee and its report.

METs and MET-minutes

A well-known physiologic effect of physical activity is that it expends energy. A metabolic equivalent, or MET, is a unit useful for describing the energy expenditure of a specific activity. A MET is the ratio of the rate of energy expended during an activity to the rate of energy expended at rest. For example, 1 MET is the rate of energy expenditure while at rest. A 4 MET activity expends 4 times the energy used by the body at rest. If a person does a 4 MET activity for 30 minutes, he or she has done $4 \times 30 = 120$ MET-minutes (or 2.0 MET-hours) of physical activity. A person could also achieve 120 MET-minutes by doing an 8 MET activity for 15 minutes.

MET-Minutes and Health Benefits

A key finding of the Advisory Committee Report is that the health benefits of physical activity depend mainly on total weekly energy expenditure due to physical activity. In scientific terms, this range is 500 to 1,000 MET-minutes per week. A range is necessary because the amount of physical activity necessary to produce health benefits cannot yet be identified with a high degree of precision; this amount varies somewhat by the health benefit. For example, activity of 500 MET-minutes a week results in a substantial reduction in the risk of premature death, but activity of more than 500 MET-minutes a week is necessary to achieve a substantial reduction in the risk of breast cancer.

Dose Response

The Advisory Committee concluded that a dose-response relationship exists between physical activity and health benefits. A range of 500 to 1,000 MET-minutes of activity per week provides substantial benefit, and amounts of activity above this range have even more benefit. Amounts of activity below this range also have some benefit. The dose-response relationship continues even within the range of 500 to 1,000 MET-minutes, in that the health benefits of 1,000 MET-minutes per week are greater than those of 500 MET-minutes per week.

Two Methods of Assessing Aerobic Intensity

The intensity of aerobic physical activity can be defined in absolute or relative terms.

Absolute Intensity

The Advisory Committee concluded that absolute moderate-intensity or vigorous-intensity physical activity is necessary for substantial health benefits, and it defined absolute aerobic intensity in terms of METs:

- Light-intensity activities are defined as 1.1 MET to 2.9 METs.

- Moderate-intensity activities are defined as 3.0 to 5.9 METs. Walking at 3.0 miles per hour requires 3.3 METs of energy expenditure and is therefore considered a moderate-intensity activity.

- Vigorous-intensity activities are defined as 6.0 METs or more. Running at 10 minutes per mile (6.0 mph) is a 10 MET activity and is therefore classified as vigorous intensity.

Relative Intensity

Intensity can also be defined relative to fitness, with the intensity expressed in terms of a percent of a person's (1) maximal heart rate, (2) heart rate reserve, or (3) aerobic capacity reserve. The Advisory Committee regarded relative moderate intensity as 40 to 59 percent of aerobic capacity reserve (where 0 percent of reserve is resting and 100 percent of reserve is maximal

effort). Relatively vigorous-intensity activity is 60 to 84 percent of reserve.

To better communicate the concept of relative intensity (or relative level of effort), the Guidelines adopted a simpler definition:

- Relatively moderate-intensity activity is a level of effort of 5 or 6 on a scale of 0 to 10, where 0 is the level of effort of sitting, and 10 is maximal effort.

- Relatively vigorous-intensity activity is a 7 or 8 on this scale.

This simplification was endorsed by the American College of Sports Medicine and the American Heart Association in their recent guidelines for older adults.[1] This approach does create a minor difference from the Advisory Committee Report definitions, however. A 5 or 6 on a 0 to 10 scale is essentially 45 percent to 64 percent of aerobic capacity reserve for moderate intensity. Similarly, a 7 or 8 on a 0 to 10 scale means 65 percent to 84 percent of reserve is the range for relatively vigorous-intensity activity.

Developing Guidelines Based on Minutes of Moderate- and Vigorous-Intensity Activity

Physical activity guidelines expressed using MET-minutes are not useful for the general public. The concept of METs is difficult to understand and few people are familiar with it. It is challenging for the public to know the MET values for all the activities they do.

As long as people who follow the Guidelines generally achieve 500 to 1,000 MET-minutes per week (or more), it is appropriate to express the Guidelines in simpler terms of minutes of moderate-intensity activity, and minutes of vigorous-intensity activity. Because not all the benefits of physical activity occur at 500 MET-minutes per week, Guidelines that help people exceed this minimum are desirable.

[1]Nelson, M. E., Rejeski, W. J., Blair, S. N., Duncan, P. W., Judge, J. O., King, A. C., et al. (2007, August). Physical activity and public health in older adults: Recommendation from the American College of Sports Medicine and the American Heart Association. *Medicine & Science in Sports & Exercise 8*, 1435–1445.

Information in the Advisory Committee Report lays the basis for expressing physical activity guidelines in minutes. The Advisory Committee indicated that 150 minutes (2 hours and 30 minutes) of moderate-intensity activity per week could be regarded as (roughly) equivalent to 500 MET-minutes per week. In fact, 3.3 METs for 150 minutes per week is equal to 500 MET-minutes per week. By recommending that adults do at least 150 minutes of moderate-intensity activity per week, adults will achieve 500 to 1,000 MET-minutes per week if the intensity is 3.3 METs or greater. As indicated by the Advisory Committee Report, people who do 150 minutes of a 3.0 to 3.2 MET activity are acceptably close to achieving 500 MET minutes. As noted earlier, walking at 3.0 miles per hour is a 3.3 MET activity. Hence, it is appropriate to communicate to the public that a "brisk walk" is walking at 3.0 miles per hour or faster.

By recommending at least 75 minutes (1 hour and 15 minutes) per week of vigorous-intensity activity, adults who choose to do vigorous-intensity activity will also generally achieve 500 to 1,000 MET-minutes per week. The lower limit of vigorous–intensity activity (6.0 METs) is twice the lower limit of moderate-intensity activity (3.0 METs). So, 75 minutes of vigorous-intensity activity per week is roughly equivalent to 150 minutes of moderate-intensity activity per week. As the MET range for vigorous-intensity activity has no upper limit, highly fit people can even exceed 1,000 MET-minutes in 75 minutes by doing activities requiring 13.4 MET or more. It is not of concern that the vigorous-intensity Guideline "misleads" people with a high degree of fitness into doing more activity than is really required to meet the Guidelines. Highly fit people have already decided to do large amounts of physical activity, as this is the only way to achieve this degree of fitness.

Finally, the Guidelines needed to address the issue that some people do both moderate-intensity and vigorous-intensity activity in a week. To determine whether they are doing enough activity to meet the Guidelines, these people need a "rule of thumb" as to how vigorous-intensity minutes substitute for moderate-intensity ones. Because 150 minutes of moderate-intensity activity and 75 minutes of vigorous-intensity activity are the minimum amounts,

the rule of thumb becomes that 1 minute of vigorous-intensity activity counts the same as 2 minutes of moderate-intensity activity.

Using Relative Intensity To Meet Guidelines Expressed in Terms of Absolute Intensity

The intent of the aerobic Guidelines for adults is to ensure that people who follow them generally achieve 500 to 1,000 MET-minutes or more. For this to occur, the definition of intensity in the Guidelines needs to be in terms of METs (i.e., absolute intensity). However, the Guidelines for Adults indicate that relative intensity can also be used as a means of assessing the intensity of aerobic activities. And the Guidelines for Older Adults *require* the use of relative intensity. How can this be appropriate?

For many adults it does not matter a great deal whether they use relative or absolute intensity. That is, following the Guidelines means they attain 500 to 1,000 MET-minutes per week using either absolute or relative intensity to guide level of effort. Their level of fitness is such that, when they do absolute moderate-intensity activities in the range of 3.0 to 5.9 METs, they generally are also doing relatively moderate-intensity activity. Similarly, absolutely vigorous and relatively vigorous activities overlap a great deal.

For adults with higher levels of fitness, using relative intensity means they will do higher amounts of activity than intended by the Guidelines. For example, a 3.5 MET activity can be relatively light for these adults, and perhaps 6.0 MET activities are relatively moderate. By doing 150 minutes of a 6.0 MET activity, they exceed the amount of activity intended in the Guideline. But this is acceptable for two reasons: First, the Guidelines encourage people to do higher amounts of activity, as higher amounts have greater health benefits. Second, people with higher levels of fitness generally can only achieve this level of fitness by doing higher amounts of activity, and thus have already chosen to do more activity.

Some adults have low levels of fitness, particularly older adults. For these adults, activities in the range of 3.0 to 5.9 METs are either relatively vigorous, or physiologically impossible. The Advisory Committee Report stated that for older adults, who commonly have low levels of fitness, the level of effort should be guided by relative intensity (as opposed to absolute). The report also stated that inactive adults should not do relatively vigorous-intensity activity when they start to increase their activity level. In other words, it is not intended or appropriate for people with low levels of fitness to meet a moderate-intensity guideline by routinely doing relatively vigorous-intensity activity.

Allowing the Use of Either Relative Intensity or Absolute Intensity in Children

The Guidelines for Children and Adolescents do not require carefully tracking of the intensity of the activity. The mix of moderate- and vigorous-intensity activity is flexible, as long as some vigorous-intensity activity is done at least 3 days per week. This flexibility means that relative and absolute intensity are both appropriate ways to track intensity.

Relative intensity is appropriate for several reasons. The exercise studies on which the Guidelines are based commonly prescribed aerobic activity using relative intensity. Children and adolescents who follow the Guidelines should have improvement in cardiorespiratory fitness, and the relative intensity of the activity is a major determinant of its fitness effects. The intent of the Advisory Committee Report is that, when a child breathes rapidly during physical activity (an indicator of relatively vigorous-intensity activity for that child), this activity should count as vigorous intensity.

However, it is not always feasible to observe children closely enough to determine their level of effort. In this case, absolute intensity can be used to judge whether the child is doing activity that counts toward the Guidelines. Brisk walking (as opposed to slow walking) counts as moderate-intensity activity, and running counts as vigorous-intensity activity, based on the typical level of effort required for these activities.

Appendix 2. Selected Examples of Injury Prevention Strategies for Common Physical Activities and Sports

This chart provides examples of various evidence-based injury prevention strategies compiled by one group of safety and injury prevention experts (Gilchrist et al., 2007). It is provided as a resource for readers and is not a product of the Physical Activity Guidelines Advisory Committee.

Activity/Sport	Proven*	Promising/Potential*
Baseball/softball	• Breakaway bases • Reduced impact balls • Faceguards/protective eyewear	• Batting helmets • Pitch count
Basketball	• Mouth guards	• Ankle disc (balance) training • Semi-rigid ankle stabilizers/braces** • Protective eyewear
Bicycling	• Helmet use[†]	• Bike paths/lanes • Retractable handle bars
Football	• Helmets and other personal protective equipment • Ankle stabilizers/braces** • Minimizing cleat length • Rule changes (no spearing, clipping, etc.) • Playing field maintenance • Preseason conditioning • Cross-training (reduce overuse injuries) • Coach training and experience	• Limiting contact during practice
Ice hockey	• Helmets with full face shield • Rule changes (fair play, no checking from behind, no high sticking, etc.) • Increased rink size	• Enforcement of rules • Discouraging fighting
In-line skating/ skateboarding	• Wrist guards • Knee/elbow pads	• Helmets
Playgrounds	• Shock-absorbing surfacing • Height standards • Maintenance standards	

Activity/Sport	Proven*	Promising/Potential*
Running/jogging	• Altered training regimen	• Shock-absorbing insoles
Skiing/snowboarding	• Training to avoid risk situations • Adjustable bindings • Wrist guards in snowboarding	• Helmets
Soccer	• Anchored, padded goal posts • Shin guards • Neuromuscular training programs[†] • Strength training	

*Proven interventions have strong evidence of effectiveness in preventing injuries. Promising/potential interventions have moderately strong evidence of effectiveness from small studies or have been tested only under laboratory conditions.

**Semi-rigid ankle stabilizers and braces have been shown to be most effective for persons with a previous history of ankle sprain. Stabilizers and braces are recommended for persons who have a previous ankle injury and are participating in all activities with a risk of ankle injury (jumping, running, twisting, etc.).

[†]Helmets worn while bicycling reduce the risk of death and injury. Educational campaigns, laws/legislation, and financial subsidy programs all increase use of helmets.

[†]Neuromuscular training programs consist of 4 elements: (1) muscle strengthening, (2) balance training, (3) jump training, and (4) learning proper mechanics (pivoting, landing, etc.).

Source: Adapted from Gilchrist, J., Saluja, G., & Marshall, S. W. (2007). Interventions to prevent sports and recreation-related injuries. In L. S. Doll, S. E. Bonzo, J. Mercy, & D. A. Sleet (Eds), *Handbook of injury and violence prevention* (pp. 117–136). New York: Springer.

Appendix 3. Federal Web Sites That Promote Physical Activity

Centers for Disease Control and Prevention (CDC)
http://www.cdc.gov/ncipc/duip/preventadultfalls.htm

Preventing Falls in Older Adults promotes physical activity as part of the approach to reducing falls and fall-related injuries among older adults.

National Institutes of Health
http://nihseniorhealth.gov/exercise/toc.html

NIH Senior Health provides aging-related health information for seniors on a variety of topics, including exercise and the causes and prevention of balance problems and falls. *Exercise and Physical Activity: Your Everyday Guide from the National Institute on Aging,* an evidence-based guide that provides information about how older adults can meet the Physical Activity Guidelines can be found at http://www.nia.nih.gov/ HealthInformation/Publications/ExerciseGuide/.

Office of the Surgeon General
http://www.surgeongeneral.gov/obesityprevention/ index.html

The Office of the Surgeon General promotes *Healthy Youth for a Healthy Future,* an HHS childhood overweight and obesity prevention initiative. The Web site provides resources to help youth stay active and make healthy choices.

President's Council on Physical Fitness and Sports
http://www.presidentschallenge.org

The President's Challenge program recognizes adults and children for meeting physical activity goals through its Presidential Active Lifestyle Award and Presidential Champions program. In addition, the program continues its longstanding physical fitness testing program for children and adolescents. An adult fitness test, found at http://www.adultfitnesstest.org, allows adults aged 18 and older to track their current level of fitness. Additional information can be found at the President's Council on Physical Fitness and Sports http://www.fitness.gov.

Division of Adolescent and School Health, CDC
http://www.cdc.gov/HealthyYouth/physicalactivity

The physical activity section of the Healthy Youth! Web site provides resources that can increase the capacity of the nation's schools to promote lifelong physical activity.

Administration on Aging (AoA)
http://www.aoa.gov/
Search: physical activity

The AoA Evidence-Based Disease Prevention Program provides examples of how community-based organizations deliver low-cost evidence-based physical activity programs that benefit older adults and help them to thrive in their communities.

Division of Nutrition, Physical Activity, and Obesity (DNPAO), CDC
http://www.cdc.gov/nccdphp/dnpa/physical/index.htm

The DNPAO physical activity Web site provides resources for program planners, health professionals, and other community members.

Federal Highway Administration
http://www.fhwa.dot.gov/environment/bikeped/index.htm

The Bicycle and Pedestrian program provides resources to help promote bicycle and pedestrian transportation use, safety, and accessibility. Resources include a listing of State Pedestrian and Bicycle Coordinators and information on funding sources and legislation. This Web site also links to the Pedestrian and Bicycle Information Center, which provides information on engineering, advocacy, education, and enforcement topics.

Environmental Protection Agency

http://www.epa.gov/aging/bhc/index.htm

The Building Healthy Communities for Active Aging program provides tools to support community efforts to employ smart growth and active aging policies and programs. One focus of the program is the Building Healthy Communities for Active Aging awards program, which recognizes communities for advancing smart growth and active aging measures.

National Institutes of Health

http://www.nhlbi.nih.gov/health/public/heart/obesity/wecan/

We Can! (Ways to Enhance Children's Activity and Nutrition) is an educational program for families and communities focused on helping youths improve food choices, increase physical activity, and reduce screen time. We Can! is jointly sponsored by the National Heart, Lung, and Blood Institute; the National Institute of Diabetes and Digestive and Kidney Diseases; the Eunice Kennedy Shriver National Institute for Child Health and Human Development; and the National Cancer Institute.

National Park Service

http://www.nps.gov/ncrc/programs/rtca/helpfultools/ht_publications.html

The Rivers, Trails, and Conservation Assistance Program has helpful tools that provide resources and information on trail and greenways programs and trail development. For example, the site has a toolbox of materials on how to turn a community dream of building a trail or revitalizing a park or open space into reality.

Health Care

U.S. Preventive Services Task Force (USPSTF)

http://www.ahrq.gov/clinic/uspstf/uspsphys.htm

The Agency for Healthcare Research & Quality supports this independent panel of experts in primary care and prevention that systematically reviews the evidence of effectiveness and develops recommendations for clinical preventive services. The USPSTF recognizes that regular physical activity helps prevent chronic disease and decrease morbidity. The USPSTF counseling recommendation about promoting physical activity is focused on behavioral counseling services delivered in primary care practices.

Worksites

Healthier Worksite Initiative, CDC

http://www.cdc.gov/nccdphp/dnpa/hwi/index.htm

This CDC initiative provides health promotion program planners working in State and Federal Government offices with information on a variety of health promotion programs, including physical activity promotion and fitness center design and management. The Web site also links to resources from other nonprofit and educational organizations through the Quick Resources section.

Be Active, Healthy, and Happy!

www.health.gov/paguidelines

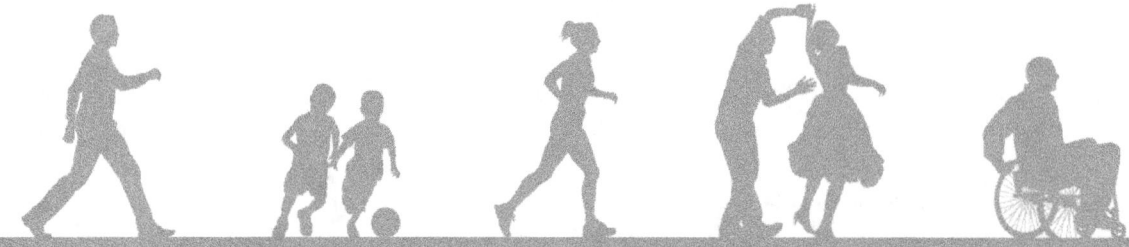

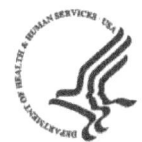 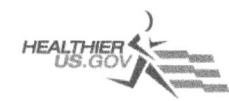

You can find more information about the new advice on physical activity at:
www.health.gov/paguidelines.

ODPHP Publication No. U0036
October 2008